ONCOLOGY: STRATEGIES FOR SUPERIOR SERVICE LINE PERFORMANCE

ECG MANAGEMENT CONSULTANTS, INC.

HealthLeaders Media
A Division of hcPro

HCPro

Oncology: Strategies for Superior Service Line Performance is published by HealthLeaders Media

Copyright © 2011 HealthLeaders Media

All rights reserved. Printed in the United States of America.   5   4   3   2   1

ISBN: 978-1-60146-866-6

No part of this publication may be reproduced, in any form or by any means, without prior written consent of HCPro, Inc., or the Copyright Clearance Center (978/750-8400). Please notify us immediately if you have received an unauthorized copy.

HCPro, Inc., provides information resources for the healthcare industry. HCPro, Inc., is not affiliated in any way with The Joint Commission, which owns the JCAHO and Joint Commission trademarks.

ECG Management Consultants, Inc., Author	Carrie Vaughan, Editor
Bob Wertz, Executive Editor	Matt Cann, Group Publisher
Doug Ponte, Cover Designer	Mike Mirabello, Senior Graphic Artist
Matt Sharpe, Production Manager	Shane Katz, Art Director
Jean St. Pierre, Senior Director of Operations	

Advice given is general. Readers should consult professional counsel for specific legal, ethical, or clinical questions.

Arrangements can be made for quantity discounts. For more information, contact:

HCPro, Inc.
75 Sylvan Street, Suite A-101
Danvers, MA 01923
Telephone: 800/650-6787 or 781/639-1872
Fax: 800/639-8511
E-mail: *customerservice@hcpro.com*

HCPro, Inc., is the parent company of HealthLeaders Media.

Visit HealthLeaders Media online at: *www.healthleadersmedia.com*

12/2011
21931

Contents

About the Authors vii

Introduction: The Evolution and Adoption of Cancer Service Lines xv

Chapter 1: Strategic Planning for Oncology Services 1

Step 1: Understanding the Content of an Oncology Strategic Plan 2
Step 2: Planning to Plan: How to Structure the Planning Process 4
Step 3: Learning About the Organization's Capabilities and the Market 9
Step 4: Identifying What the Organization Wants to Accomplish 16
Step 5: Making It Happen 20
Key Takeaways 29

Chapter 2: Creating a Successful Oncology Service Line 31

Introduction to Service Line Principles 32
Key Elements for Service Line Success 34
Implementation Issues 50
The Future for Oncology Service Lines 52
Key Takeaways 53

Contents

Chapter 3: The Importance of Governance and Leadership 55

Oncology Governance Structures 55
Oncology Service Line Leadership 67
Managing Performance..72
Key Takeaways 75

Chapter 4: Creating Aligned Physician Relationships..........................77

Affiliation Models 78
Physician Alignment Planning Process 102
Key Takeaways 107

Chapter 5: Key Elements of a Successful Oncology Transaction 109

Definition of the Transaction Goals..110
Evaluate Business Implications 111
Development of the Organizational Structure...116
Developing a Compensation Plan 118
Implementation 131
Key Takeaways 134

Chapter 6: Navigating the Challenges of Oncology Reimbursement 137

Keys to Oncology Reimbursement: Legislation, Drugs, Professional Fees............139
Implications for Hospitals 153
Other Reimbursement Trends...166
Key Takeaways 169

Chapter 7: Clinical Integration and the Oncology Care Model 173

Coordinating Cancer Care: The Importance of the Navigator Role 174
New Approach to Treatment Planning: Multidisciplinary Care 178
CAM 192
Key Takeaways 195

Chapter 8: Academic Cancer Centers 197

Three Game Changers for Academic Cancer Centers 198
Keys to Success in Academic Oncology 201
Streamlined Leadership Structure 202
Alignment of Financial Interests 211
Key Takeaways 221

Chapter 9: Maximizing Clinical Research Operations 223

Research Overview 224
Best Practices in Research Program Planning 226
Why Billing for Clinical Trials Is So Complex 233
The Nuts and Bolts of Billing for Clinical Trials 239
The Last Step: Audit Process and Performance 243
Key Takeaways 244

Appendix A: Sample Interview Guide 247

Appendix B: Internal and External Assessment Key Analyses 253

About the Authors

Jessica L. Turgon

Jessica L. Turgon has 15 years of experience in cancer center strategic planning, operations improvement, and revenue cycle optimization. She leads the oncology practice and is a senior manager at ECG Management Consultants, Inc.'s (ECG) oncology practice, and has extensive experience developing and leading oncology programs in both community and academic settings. Turgon's project work has helped several cancer centers realize significant revenue and efficiency gains while also improving patient and staff satisfaction. Turgon has spoken to oncology organizations, as well as authored articles on clinical trial operations, reimbursement strategies, and operational improvements in oncology service line development. Prior to joining ECG, Turgon was the administrative leader for several National Cancer Institute–designated comprehensive cancer centers. She received a master of business administration degree from George Washington University and a bachelor of arts degree in political science from Marymount University.

Matthew R. Sturm

Since joining ECG, in 2003, **Matthew R. Sturm** has assisted dozens of organizations with strategic and operational issues related to their oncology programs, including feasibility assessments for new modalities, financial planning, physician

About the Authors

compensation planning, service line planning, joint venture development, physician practice acquisition, and the formation and expansion of clinical research programs. Sturm, who is a senior manager at ECG, has particular knowledge and expertise regarding the 340B Drug Pricing Program and radiation oncology. He is a regular speaker at the Association of Community Cancer Centers conferences and has written a number of articles on related subjects. In addition, Sturm serves on the expert advisory panel for *Oncology Issues*, the journal of the Association of Community Cancer Centers. Sturm holds a master of business administration degree from Indiana University's Kelley School of Business and a bachelor of arts degree in biology from Baylor University.

Christopher T. Collins

Christopher T. Collins is a principal in the academic healthcare practice and works with boards and executive leadership of academic medical centers (AMC), health systems, and large physician organizations in the areas of strategy, health system development and partnerships, and clinical program development. Collins is often called upon to lead joint planning efforts between the hospital/health system and physician organizations to achieve an integrated model of care that effectively aligns the entities' strategic, financial, and operational interests. At a program level, his specialty areas include cancer, cardiovascular, and neurosciences. Collins is a frequent author and presenter on issues such as AMC integration and hospital/physician alignment. He holds a master's degree in healthcare administration from the George Washington University.

About the Authors

Darin E. Libby

As a senior manager and a member of ECG's healthcare practice, **Darin E. Libby** has worked extensively with health system, hospital, and medical group clients to address a variety of planning, business development, and operational issues. Prior to joining ECG, he worked at Overlake Hospital Medical Center in Bellevue, WA, where he led an effort to build a new hospital and managed the physician practice division, which included select cancer specialists. In addition, Libby served as the cancer service line administrator at The Methodist Hospital in Houston. He received a master of health administration degree from Washington University School of Medicine in St. Louis and a bachelor of arts degree from Austin College.

Kathryn K. Reed

Kathryn K. Reed, a manager at ECG, has broad experience in strategic planning, financial analysis, service line development, hospital/physician alignment, and transactions. She has expertise in oncology services and has worked with a variety of clients on their service line and programmatic needs. Most recently, Reed facilitated several hospital/physician transactions, including the acquisition of an independent oncology group. She has substantial experience developing alignment models, designing funds flow and governance structures, conducting fair market value assessments, evaluating the 340B Drug Pricing Program and provider-based conversions, supporting physician practice valuations, facilitating hospital/physician negotiations, and providing ongoing integration assistance. Reed holds a master of business administration degree from the University of Washington Michael G. Foster School of Business and a bachelor of science degree in biology from The University of Texas at Austin.

About the Authors

Jason S. Rife

Jason S. Rife, a manager at ECG, joined the consultancy in 2006 and has nearly 10 years of consulting experience with an extensive background in clinical operations, organizational performance, oncology revenue enhancement, human capital, and healthcare policy. He has implemented organizational and operational strategies for large healthcare organizations and has developed human resources strategies. Rife has a master of public health degree in health policy and management from Columbia University and a bachelor of arts degree in political science from Yale University.

Gregory P. Silva

As a manager in ECG's Boston office, **Gregory P. Silva** has focused on strategy and business planning, including multidisciplinary institute/service line development, hospital/physician arrangements, and faculty group practice/physician practice assessments. He is actively involved in the firm's oncology practice and has assisted numerous clients with oncology service line development and related practice transactions. Silva holds a master of business administration degree from Boston University Graduate School of Management and a bachelor of science degree in health policy and management from Providence College.

Contributing Authors

ECG's Oncology Affinity Group is responsible for the thought leadership and knowledge development of the firm's oncology practice. The group has extensive

About the Authors

experience in strategic planning, operations improvement, hospital/physician transactions, and reimbursement optimization in oncology services. In addition to the authors, key contributions were made by the following members of the group:

- **James P. Donohue, senior manager,** has more than 17 years of experience in the healthcare industry working with major medical centers, with a focus on business operations and strategic planning, oncology reimbursement strategies, and contracting.

- **Krista L. Fakoory, manager,** has extensive experience in operations and process improvement, genetic and disease research, and business development. Fakoory has assisted in the development of oncology service line management and governance structures, performed fair market value assessments, and participated in strategic planning for clinical research programs.

- **Kevin P. Forster, principal,** has a strong track record of implementing innovative solutions in cancer specialties that foster integration among organizations, services, and clinical programs. Forster's most recent client experience includes developing several hospital/physician joint ventures, designing integration plans for hospital-employed physicians, and performing multidisciplinary service line planning for oncology and other specialties.

- **Jada L. Keith, senior consultant,** has assisted hospital and medical group clients with service line strategic planning, fair market valuations, joint venture development, and physician compensation planning. Most recently, Keith assisted a community hospital system and a multispecialty medical group with their joint oncology service line planning efforts.

About the Authors

- **Kevin M. Kennedy, principal,** has assisted dozens of hospitals, health systems, and medical groups with solving their strategic, financial, and operational problems. Kennedy has particular expertise in strategic planning, cancer service line development, and hospital/physician relationships. He is a frequent speaker before industry associations and is a past recipient of the Yerger/Seawell Article of the Year award for outstanding contribution to professional literature from the Healthcare Financial Management Association.

- **Stephen F. Messinger, principal,** has worked with a broad range of healthcare organizations and has assisted hospitals, health systems, and physician groups in cancer strategy development and performance improvement. Messinger has led large oncology transactions and service line development projects.

- **Katherine Collings Ray, senior consultant,** has assisted community hospital and medical group clients in evaluating and implementing the 340B Drug Pricing Program and determining optimal alignment structures in oncology specialties.

- **Malita I. Scott, manager,** has focused her career on oncology service line development and operations improvement. Scott has served as project manager for the development of new multidisciplinary cancer institutes, assisted with the completion of numerous operational improvement initiatives in hospitals and physician practice settings, performed multiple compensation planning and fair market value assessments, and evaluated clinical research programs for adherence to regulatory and financial guidelines.

About ECG

ECG offers a broad range of strategic-, financial-, operational-, and technology-related consulting services to healthcare providers. As a leader in the industry, ECG provides specialized expertise to community hospitals, academic medical centers, health systems, and medical groups. For nearly 40 years, its more than 110 consultants have played an instrumental role in developing and implementing innovative and customized solutions that effectively address issues confronting healthcare providers. ECG has offices in Boston, San Diego, San Francisco, Seattle, St. Louis, and Washington, DC.

At the heart of its expertise in oncology services is an understanding of the competencies needed to differentiate top-performing oncology service lines. ECG has had the pleasure of working with premier oncology programs, helping hospitals and physicians work together to build and develop service line strategies and structures.

INTRODUCTION

The Evolution and Adoption of Cancer Service Lines

In the four decades since President Richard Nixon announced a "total national commitment for the conquest of cancer" while signing into law the National Cancer Act, incredible progress has been made in understanding the fundamental nature of cancer and translating those findings into prevention and treatment of the disease. The result has been a dramatic increase in the likelihood of survival for cancer patients and a better quality of life for survivors. Since the 1970s, cancer survival rates have improved significantly (see Figure A), resulting in an estimated 898,000 fewer cancer deaths during the period of 1991 through 2007.[1]

Although these developments have been nothing short of remarkable, cancer remains the second leading cause of death in the United States (see Figure B), and cancer incidence is expected to increase sharply over the next 20 years as the U.S. population continues to grow and age.[2]

Research has also shed light on the complex nature of cancer. In fact, it is no longer possible to discuss cancer as a single disease, but as a collection of "more than 200 diseases—all of which have different causes and require different treatments."[3]

Introduction: The Evolution and Adoption of Cancer Service Lines

FIGURE A
TRENDS IN FIVE-YEAR RELATIVE SURVIVAL RATE

Tumor Site	1975 to 1977	1999 to 2006
Breast (female)	75%	90%
Colon	52%	66%
Leukemia	36%	55%
Lung and bronchus	13%	16%
Melanoma	83%	93%
Non-Hodgkin's lymphoma	48%	69%
Ovary	37%	45%
Pancreas	3%	6%
Prostate	69%	100%
Rectum	49%	69%
Urinary bladder	74%	81%
All sites	50%	68%

Source: American Cancer Society. (2011). *Cancer Facts & Figures 2011*. Atlanta: American Cancer Society.

The Players

The same complexity that defines cancer at a molecular level is reflected in the array of specialists and healthcare providers required to treat patients, as well as the business models required to bring these disparate providers together to function as a cohesive unit. Typically, oncology providers belong to multiple,

FIGURE B
UNITED STATES LEADING CAUSES OF DEATH—2007

Rank	Cause of Death	2007 Annual Number of Deaths	Percentage of All Deaths—2007
1.	Heart disease	616,067	25.4%
2.	Cancer	562,875	23.2%
3.	Cerebrovascular disease	135,952	5.6%
4.	Chronic lower respiratory disease	127,924	5.3%
5.	Accidents (unintentional injuries)	123,706	5.1%
6.	Alzheimer's disease	74,632	3.1%
7.	Diabetes mellitus	71,382	2.9%
8.	Influenza and pneumonia	52,717	2.2%
9.	Nephritis	46,448	1.9%
10.	Septicemia	34,828	1.4%

Source: National Center for Health Statistics, Centers for Disease Control and Prevention. (2010). *U.S. Mortality Data 2007.* Atlanta: Centers for Disease Control and Prevention.

independently operating entities, each with their own, often competing, clinical, financial, and political concerns. This disparity among providers results in complicated relationships between individual providers and organizations, making coordination of care especially difficult. Figure C explores several key characteristics of each type of provider involved in the oncology treatment team.

Introduction: The Evolution and Adoption of Cancer Service Lines

FIGURE C
THE ONCOLOGY TREATMENT TEAM: KEY CHARACTERISTICS

Specialty/Service	Description	Practice Overview	Referral Patterns	Power/Influence on Team
Medical oncology	• Medical specialty that concentrates on oncology treatment with medications (e.g., chemotherapy, analgesics, hormones)	• Most care is delivered in an outpatient setting • Chemotherapy infusions represent both a key treatment modality and income source • Thereby, medical oncologists are exposed to risks associated with Medicare's decreasing reimbursement for medications and high drug costs* • Increasingly, private practices are transitioning to hospital employment given changes in reimbursement	Often thought of as the oncology coordinator of care ("gatekeeper"); in reality, they are not exclusively gatekeepers	• High • Medical oncologists oversee patient care from diagnosis through treatment and often beyond as managers of survivorship care.

FIGURE C
THE ONCOLOGY TREATMENT TEAM: KEY CHARACTERISTICS (CONT.)

Specialty/Service	Description	Practice Overview	Referral Patterns	Power/Influence on Team
Surgical oncology	• Surgical specialty with clinical experience concentrated in tumor excisions • Surgical subspecialization includes breast, cardiothoracic, neurology, and gastroenterology, among others	• The majority of surgical oncology services are provided in a hospital setting • Historically, a higher percentage of surgeons were employed by hospitals than other oncology subspecialties	Surgical oncologists are key referral sources for radiation oncology; referrals to surgical oncology may come from a variety of sources	• Medium • Surgical oncology patients will typically require other oncology services and treatment for comorbidities, so the surgeons are important members of the oncology team

FIGURE C
THE ONCOLOGY TREATMENT TEAM: KEY CHARACTERISTICS (CONT.)

Specialty/Service	Description	Practice Overview	Referral Patterns	Power/Influence on Team
Radiation oncology	• Medical specialty that uses radiation therapy in the treatment of cancer	• Most care is delivered in an outpatient setting • Radiation therapy requires a significant financial investment in technology (e.g., linear accelerator), but in return, it is also the driver of revenue • Radiation oncologists are exposed to risks associated with Medicare's trend in decreasing reimbursement for their services**	Typically, radiation oncologists account for limited referrals to other clinicians	• Medium • Radiation oncologists often play a smaller role in program building/development than do medical or surgical oncologists • However, technical income from radiation oncology is often used to support other elements of the oncology program, making the service clinically, financially, and strategically important to the program

FIGURE C
THE ONCOLOGY TREATMENT TEAM: KEY CHARACTERISTICS (CONT.)

Specialty/ Service	Description	Practice Overview	Referral Patterns	Power/Influence on Team
Support services	Interdisciplinary patient care often includes a variety of nonallopathic services, such as nutrition education, physical therapy, occupational therapy, and social worker counseling	• Services may be provided to inpatients and outpatients • Providing the support services alone is typically not financially viable because they may not be eligible for payer reimbursement	Support services are dependent on referrals from physicians	• Low • Support services typically have the least influence on the oncology team

FIGURE C
THE ONCOLOGY TREATMENT TEAM: KEY CHARACTERISTICS (CONT.)

Specialty/ Service	Description	Practice Overview	Referral Patterns	Power/Influence on Team
Diagnostic services	• *Imaging* – Technology used to identify and assess a patient's condition. Modalities include x-ray, CT scan, MRI, ultrasound, and nuclear medicine • *Laboratory* – Studies performed to assist in the management of patient care, such as blood diagnostics and pathology reports	• Imaging and laboratory services are provided to inpatients and outpatients • Reimbursement for imaging services is currently being heavily scrutinized and will likely experience further reductions	Diagnostic services are dependent on referrals from physicians	• Low • Diagnostic services do not directly manage a patient's therapeutic regimen, but they are essential to comprehensive, multidisciplinary care and programmatic economic viability

* See Chapter 6 for more discussion on Medicare reimbursement changes.
** For example, there have been recent Medicare changes to the radiation oncology practice expense methodology. See Chapter 6 for more reimbursement trends.

Source: ECG Management Consultants, Inc.

Introduction: The Evolution and Adoption of Cancer Service Lines

Given the nature of the disease (or, more appropriately, diseases) and the challenges associated with bringing together a diverse group of providers, it is not surprising that the market for oncology services is, more often than not, characterized by inconsistent access to care, limited coordination among providers, frequent variability in treatment, and redundancy/waste in the system due to the provision of duplicative services. At the same time, payers, most notably Medicare, struggle with how to cover the rising costs of cancer care. In recent years, Medicare has adopted strategies to both provide immediate savings (e.g., cutting payments to providers) and longer-term systematic change through a number of innovative payment mechanisms (e.g., accountable care organizations, bundled payments, pay for performance).

The Programs

The evolution of the oncology payment model is leading many healthcare organizations to transform the oncology care model in their communities by offering more coordinated and comprehensive services that provide high quality for patients and high value to payers. Many hospitals are developing oncology service line structures that have the potential to improve clinical and financial performance, encourage physician involvement, create a distinct brand in the market, and ultimately gain a competitive advantage. While implementation of an oncology service line varies widely among hospitals, there is broad agreement that this type of is necessary for success.

Based on decades of work with a wide range of oncology providers, from small private practices to National Cancer Institute–designated cancer centers, our

Introduction: The Evolution and Adoption of Cancer Service Lines

experience indicates that successful oncology service lines typically share the following characteristics:

- **Facility and identity:** The service line has a facility or center where all cancer services can be presented to patients in a coordinated manner. The service line also has a brand name and image that is identifiable by patients and physicians in the community.

- **Coordination:** Clinical services are delivered seamlessly throughout the continuum of cancer care. As patients progress through each phase of treatment, providers share information to better inform the course of treatment, prevent unnecessary duplication of services, and ensure adherence to evidence-based oncology practice guidelines across different specialties and sites of service.

- **Clinical programs:** Differentiation occurs through the development of multidisciplinary tumor-site–specific programs, typically focusing on one, or all, of the most common cancer tumor sites (i.e., breast or lung). A fully developed clinical program operates with dedicated staff and support resources and is often marketed as a featured component of the oncology program. In order to provide tumor-specific expertise, successful programs attract providers who are highly qualified and experienced in treating tumor-specific cancer sites.

- **Clinical trials:** Clinical trials enable patients to have access to treatment options that may be beneficial but are still in experimental phases. A robust research program may be a key asset to recruiting both patients and clinicians to the program.

Introduction: The Evolution and Adoption of Cancer Service Lines

- **Support services:** A full range of psychosocial support services (e.g., patient navigation, mental health and social work, financial counseling) are offered to complement diagnostic and treatment services. These services are integral to the provision of high-quality patient care, and leading programs are those able to proactively identify and match patients to the services offered.

- **Technology:** State-of-the-art technology is used in the diagnosis and treatment of patients. This includes the implementation of electronic medical records and health information exchanges, which facilitate the flow of clinical information and enhance decision-making among providers.

- **Access:** Services are easily accessible and provided in a patient-centric setting. Colocating a range of diagnostic, treatment, and support services improves access and provides physical and psychological benefits to patients.

- **Physician governance:** Well-performing oncology programs have a well-defined physician governance organization that incorporates physicians into policy and strategy setting activities, enabling the physicians to have a meaningful role in charting the direction for the program.

The remainder of this book provides details regarding the creation and operation of a successful oncology service line. The content of the chapters was designed to allow quick access to topics of special interest to the reader.

Introduction: The Evolution and Adoption of Cancer Service Lines

References

1. American Cancer Society. (2011). *Cancer Facts & Figures 2011.* Atlanta: American Cancer Society.

2. American Association for Cancer Research. (2011). *Cancer Progress Report 2011: Transforming Patient Care Through Innovation.* Philadelphia: American Association for Cancer Research.

3. Ibid.

CHAPTER 1

Strategic Planning for Oncology Services

Oncology has emerged as a critical service line for virtually all hospitals and health systems, so it is not surprising that significant investments are being made to bolster oncology services and expand market share. Much of the investment in oncology, however, is done with minimal planning and little thought about the long-term goals of the institution. For example, based on aspirations to grow patient volume, a hospital may decide that it needs to expand and update its infusion center. A business plan is prepared that demonstrates an acceptable return on investment, and the project moves forward. The problem is that important considerations are often missing, such as how this fits into the broader need for oncology services, how the project or service will be coordinated with other oncology services, options for expansion (e.g., a separate site or partnership with an existing provider), and whether this is a priority investment as compared to other opportunities.

In short, is this decision consistent with the long-term cancer strategy of the organization? Unfortunately, most hospitals cannot answer this question because they lack an explicit strategy for oncology services. This chapter lays out the basics of an effective cancer strategy, including the following five-step process:

Chapter 1

1. Understanding the content of an oncology strategic plan

2. Planning to plan: How to structure the site planning process

3. Learning about the organization's capabilities and the market

4. Identifying what the organization wants to accomplish

5. Making it happen

Step 1: Understanding the Content of an Oncology Strategic Plan

A successful strategic plan is built upon three distinct characteristics:

1. **Focus**—What the hospital does and does not do in pursuit of its objectives to provide market-leading services to patients and physicians

2. **Differentiation**—How the hospital creates value for patients and physicians in a way that is different from its competitors

3. **Fit**—The unique combination of activities that leverages the hospital's strengths and locks out competitors

Ultimately, strategic planning is a resource prioritization and allocation process. The hospital must decide where the most potential gain exists and where the organization needs and desires to focus both its financial and human resources. By creating an oncology strategy, hospital leadership has taken an important step in making oncology services a focal point of the hospital, and the strategic planning process should result in an improvement in both the organization's competitive position and financial situation. A key role of the strategic planning process is the development of consensus among the organization's stakeholders regarding how future success will be measured, monitored, and achieved.

A fundamental aspect for the development of a cancer services strategy is a clear progression from vision to goals to strategies to tactics. The vision and goals set the direction and guide how the oncology program ultimately serves its patients, physicians, staff, and community. Developing a program vision up front is an essential part of establishing an oncology program that has a sustainable advantage, meaning a program that is focused, differentiated, and competitive. From the vision and goals come the strategies, which form the framework of the initiatives to be achieved in pursuit of the vision. The tactics describe in more granular terms how the strategies will be achieved and pave the way for implementation planning. This strategic planning framework is depicted in Figure 1.1.

For a strategic plan to be successful, it should be driven by a clear and compelling vision and direction. At the same time, an effective strategic planning process needs to result in practical and actionable strategies and tactics. It should provide the overall direction needed to focus the organization's efforts and resources, as well as produce the implementable actions needed to ensure that the identified strategic direction can be achieved.

Chapter 1

FIGURE 1.1
STRATEGIC PLANNING FRAMEWORK

Vision determines the overall direction of service line development.

Goals are specific results that the program hopes to achieve within the next 12 to 24 months.

Strategy is the formulation of an approach for allocating resources to accomplish the goals of the organization.

Tactics are the set of actions that reinforce the overall strategy and interact to create a strong "fit" in the market.

Source: ECG Management Consultants, Inc.

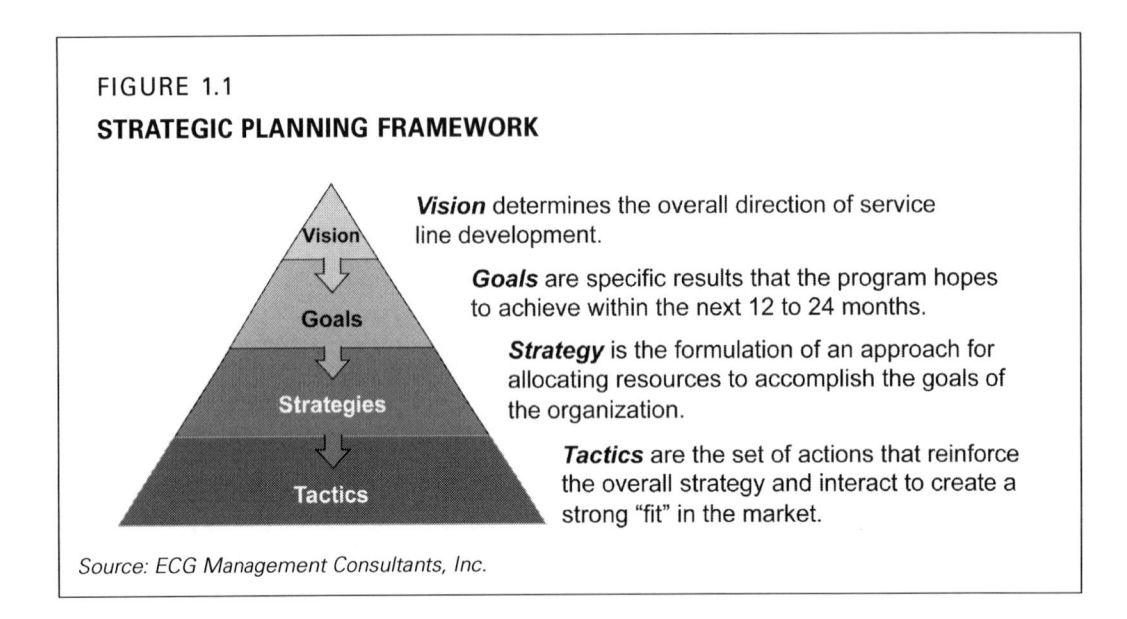

Step 2: Planning to Plan: How to Structure the Planning Process

Creating an effective oncology strategic plan is a complex process that should be spelled out in advance and understood by all participants. Hospitals need to secure the participation of diverse stakeholders, ensure that the stakeholders' time is spent wisely, and clearly identify the timelines and outcomes that are expected of key stakeholders. Typically the use of a steering committee, coupled with a work plan for the creation of a strategy, is a very useful tool.

The steering committee

A successful oncology strategy cannot be developed solely by hospital management. It should involve all key stakeholders in the process so that broad commitment and support across the organization is developed. It is far better to work out

Strategic Planning for Oncology Services

the contentious political, operational, and financial issues during the planning process rather than create a plan that cannot be implemented.

The use of a steering committee can ensure that key individuals are deeply involved in the process. The steering committee guiding the oncology strategic planning process should include hospital leadership as well as physicians. Typically a steering committee of 12 or fewer members is most efficient in terms of size. Steering committee members from the hospital typically include the following:

- Oncology manager/director

- Director of the employed physician practice (if applicable)

- Chief operating officer or CEO

- Representatives from finance and planning

- Nursing leader

To ensure inclusive representation from the medical staff, be sure to include physicians from key specialties, including the medical directors or key community specialists such as:

- Medical oncology

- Radiation oncology

- Surgical oncology

Chapter 1

- Gynecologists

- Urologists

Given the complexity of the oncology community (number of physicians, differing clinical backgrounds, various employment arrangements, etc.), some programs have found it beneficial to start the planning process with a subset of cancer specialists. Often, medical oncology is viewed as the backbone of the program; therefore, some organizations have started with a medical oncology planning group and then added other specialties as the process gained traction and direction. Regardless, it is important to fashion the steering committee membership to the unique needs of each political environment.

When considering which physicians to include on the steering committee, part of the decision should be based on who is seen as an opinion leader by the medical staff. Ideally, the physicians should also be able to "wear two hats" and constructively participate in the process to advance not just their practice, but the oncology service as a whole. Ultimately, part of the role of the physician participants is to sell the strategic plan to their colleagues throughout the process. After creating the steering committee, other stakeholders can be involved via focus groups, interviews and/or participation in select meetings, and involvement in task force or subcommittee activity as appropriate.

SAMPLE MEETING PLAN

Meeting 1—Discuss project work plan and objectives

- Finalize project scope and summarize project work plan and objectives
- Seek steering committee member feedback

Meeting 2—Review market assessment and key interview findings

- Present results of market assessment and key interview findings
- Discuss implications of the assessment

Meeting 3—Draft service line vision, goals, and structures

- Discuss working vision and potential service line leadership structures
- Define service line goals

Meeting 4—Develop strategic initiatives and finalize service line structures

- Finalize working vision and preferred leadership structures
- Discuss oncology service line vision and goals
- Develop and evaluate strategies
- Facilitate discussion, prioritization, and selection of initiatives
- Discuss tactical plan

Meeting 5—Finalize strategies and review business plan

- Present finalized strategies and business plan
- Discuss implementation timeline and designate accountabilities

Chapter 1

The work plan

Developing a work plan at the outset of the project ensures that the process is structured and transparent. It provides participants with a road map of the steps needed to develop the plan. Given that the steering committee members include busy physicians and key leaders within the hospital, it is important for them to understand how their time is going to be used, as well as the timeline from vision development to implementation planning.

Typically, four to five meetings of the steering committee are needed to complete the planning process. The number of meetings varies depending on the magnitude of changes being considered and the organizational culture. If the organization is contemplating transformational strategies, such as retooling the physician leadership structure or creating new programs, more meetings will likely be needed to discuss all implications, weigh the financial impact, and reach consensus. Similarly, the culture at each organization is different, and the process of facilitating the steering committee to reach a decision is unique to each hospital culture, and may take more or fewer meetings, depending on the amount of discussion needed. An overview of the typical strategic planning process for an oncology service line is presented Figure 1.2.

Strategic Planning for Oncology Services

FIGURE 1.2
STRATEGIC PLANNING PROCESS

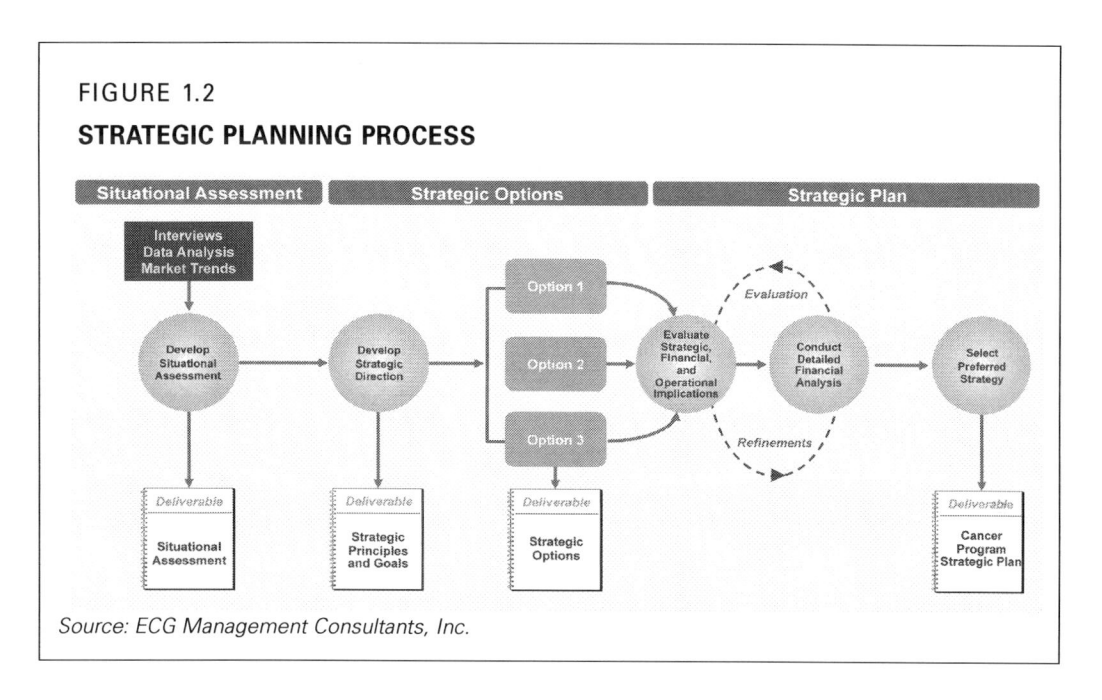

Source: ECG Management Consultants, Inc.

Step 3: Learning About the Organization's Capabilities and the Market

After the steering committee and work plan have been developed, the next step is to take a close look at the organization and the market. During this step, commonly referred to as a situational assessment, the organization will develop a comprehensive picture of its current oncology program and current position in the market, as well as the opportunities and challenges that it may face going forward. To gain the needed level of understanding, it is necessary to look at the oncology program from both a quantitative and qualitative perspective. The key components of the situational assessment include interview findings; internal and external assessments; and a strengths, weaknesses, opportunities, and threats (SWOT) analysis that details key

Chapter 1

implications to the strategic planning process. Each of these components is described in detail in this chapter.

The interview process

Interviews are an excellent way to ensure that the variety of perspectives on key issues is understood and that each participant has input into the planning process. Interviews provide an interactive forum for gathering information and are particularly effective if they are conducted by a third party to allow for confidentiality and create an environment where participants feel free to openly share their viewpoints. Whether interviewing an outside consultant or a member of administration who is not intimately involved in the service, the interviewer needs to be able to create an environment where those being interviewed feel free to voice their true opinions.

The goal of the interview process is to reveal areas of agreement, disagreement, and potential confusion. Key themes emerge concerning the potential direction for the service and critical issues that need resolution.

Who should be interviewed?

Interviews are the time to gain a wide perspective of the current oncology service and key stakeholders' vision for the service in the future. Therefore, interviewing a broad base of individuals is important. Steering committee members and senior hospital leadership should be interviewed—they will provide perspective on how the oncology service fits into their overall vision for the hospital, as well as input on any sensitive areas that should be given special consideration as part of the strategic planning process. Managers of key areas, including departmental heads and nursing leaders, can provide an on-the-ground perspective of some of the operational challenges that are currently being faced, as well as potential resource requirements. Physicians from diverse constituencies, which may be from multiple physician groups and diverse specialties, should be included. Their input is helpful not only in understanding their goals and concerns, but also in garnering information about patient care trends and referral patterns.

Two additional stakeholders should be considered for interview: competitors and payers. Competitors include other hospitals in the service area and physicians who refer to or exclusively use a competitor. They are often surprisingly open to sharing perspectives, plans, and concerns. Payers are increasingly important in terms of interest and opportunities for value-based reimbursement and the use of best practices that can be a competitive advantage. In all, depending on the size and complexity of the program, 20–35 interviews may be necessary.

A sample physician interview guide is included in Appendix A to demonstrate what should be included in the interview, including the breadth and depth of the subjects explored. Questions can easily be retooled to be appropriate for interviews for nonphysician stakeholders.

Collecting and analyzing data

Effective strategic planning will require looking at how the hospital's oncology program has grown and changed over time, as well as how it ranks compared to competitors' programs. Gathering and analyzing data is important to ground planning in facts, rather than assumptions, and to accurately assess the potential for growth in oncology services over time. However, a key limitation to a quantitative market assessment for oncology services is the dearth of publicly available

Chapter 1

market data (e.g., number of radiation treatments), because the majority of services are provided on an ambulatory basis, frequently in nonhospital-owned venues. Given this trend, many programs rely on tumor registry data and industry benchmarks to size the market and extrapolate market share.

Internal and external assessments—key analyses

Typically, the internal assessment looks at volume, financial performance, operational efficiency, and quality/outcomes for the oncology program over the past few years. Analyzing three years of data can help identify trends and the impact of key initiatives. The following are three tips to keep in mind when analyzing internal data for the oncology program:

1. It is important to note that oncology presents a unique challenge in accurately identifying the patient population. Due to the prevalence of comorbidities among the oncology patient population, cancer may not be the primary diagnosis.

2. Because the preponderance of cancer care is rendered in an outpatient setting, caution should be exercised to avoid relying too heavily on findings from an analysis of inpatient data.

3. Given the limited access to outpatient data, mapping oncology services provided/available within the network and identifying who provides them can be a valuable exercise to size the current program, compare it against competitors, and identify potential service gaps.

The external assessment provides insight into what the competition is doing and what differentiates the oncology program within key service areas. This assessment requires defining the market geographically and then identifying the key competitors within the market. (An outline of typical analyses performed to identify internal and external trends is included in Appendix B.)

Putting it all together

The final task of any situational assessment is developing an understanding of what has been learned from the interview and data collection process. Whether this takes the form of a SWOT analysis or a summary of key findings, it is important to highlight the key takeaways in order to make sense of the data and provide insight into critical factors that should be evaluated as the effectiveness of potential strategies is examined. See Figure 1.3 for an illustration of the classic four-square SWOT analysis.

Chapter 1

FIGURE 1.3

SAMPLE SWOT ANALYSIS

Strengths	Weaknesses
• Quality of care provided • Skill of physicians • Strong hospital leadership and its commitment to service line development • Inception of the women's health program • Efficient patient transfers within the system • Strong presence in the market	• Lack of clear strategic direction for service line • Limited oncology infrastructure within hospital system • Fragmented care delivery model with limited coordination • Conflicting/competitive financial interests between hospital and physicians
Opportunities	**Threats**
• Work more collaboratively with the surgeons and other disciplines (e.g., tumor boards) • Continue to develop physician leadership and governance • Patient demand for an integrated care delivery model • Develop a more integrated oncology program within the system • Promote oncology infrastructure through marketing and communication efforts • Enhance clinical coordination through the development of a navigation program or multidisciplinary cancer clinics • Create a common patient experience	• Key competitors becoming more aggressive • Reimbursement climate changing the physician practice dynamics • Physician groups forming an affiliation with another program

Source: ECG Management Consultants, Inc.

SAMPLE WORKING VISION

Patient-focused care:

- We will excel at delivering high-quality, safe, and patient-centered care

- Physicians, other clinical staff, and administration will work together to ensure that services will be organized and delivered in a manner that ensures the best patient experience possible

- Each provider will strive to coordinate the delivery of services in a way that achieves optimal access to care, quality of care, personalized attention, and cost of providing care

- We will be recognized as a leader in healthcare quality, as demonstrated by national certifications, adherence to clinical pathways, and demonstrable clinical outcomes

Programmatic growth:

- The program will continue to serve the local community as it expands its geographic reach in order to build volumes, develop subspecialty areas of expertise, and enhance financial performance

- The program will build stronger relationships with referring physicians as well as create a brand that is differentiated in the minds of patients and referring physicians

- The program will be viewed by patients and providers as a destination center

Comprehensive program scope:

- The hospital remains committed to enhancing its regional leadership position in oncology services by offering the breadth of services needed to both meet the needs of oncology patients and differentiate itself in the market

Chapter 1

> **SAMPLE WORKING VISION (CONT.)**
>
> - We will expand the mix of services offered (e.g., ENT, urology) to ensure that the program is comprehensive in scope
>
> Team-driven, coordinated care:
>
> - The oncology program builds a collaborative work environment among providers to reinforce the culture of success
>
> - The oncology program continues to develop standard protocols and processes in the inpatient and ambulatory setting
>
> - The hospital and the physicians demonstrate respect for and responsibility to each other
>
> - The providers' desire to help the oncology program succeed is supported by their shared goals, strong work ethic, and dedication to the growth of their practices
>
> - The collaborative team approach allows for the development of a well-respected, powerful, and unified brand

Step 4: Identifying What the Organization Wants to Accomplish

At the foundation of any strategic plan is the vision for the organization's future. The organizational vision acts as a touchstone to guide leadership and the strategic planning effort. While the traditional one-line hospital vision statement can be important as a concise, easily communicated and remembered statement of desired direction, it is limited in its power to describe the nuances of a complicated situation. In contrast, a working vision is a descriptive statement detailing four to six tenets that will guide management over the next five years. The benefit of taking a narrative form is that it is able to capture all key elements and paint a picture of the vision for the organization. The best visions are endorsed by all key stakeholders—the perspectives of administration, physicians, staff, and even patients are contained within it, making the vision meaningful for everyone with a stake in the hospital's future.

Developing goals

Goals should be explicit accomplishments that the organization intends to achieve within a given time frame based on its vision of the future. It is often useful to convert the information gathered from interviews, data collection, and the vision creation process into a goals grid. The grid is useful in identifying not only what the organization wants to enhance or create, but also what it should delete or avoid (Figure 1.4 illustrates the format and content of a goals grid).

Chapter 1

FIGURE 1.4
SAMPLE GOALS GRID

	Has	Does Not Have
Wants	**Preserve** • Clinical expertise • Quality of patient care • Program size and market presence • Strong reputation as part of the community • Shared responsibility for success of the program • Personalized attention to patients • Healthy physician/staff relationships • Strong, consensus-building hospital leadership • Strong nursing program	**Achieve** • Quality outcomes and growth in volumes • More successful recruiting and retaining of new physicians • Comprehensive program scope • Tumor site programs and clinical research • New facilities with consolidated services and multidisciplinary clinics • Institutional partnerships • National recognition • Shared governance structure • Streamline decision-making • Access to innovative technology
Does Not Want	**Eliminate** • Scheduling and patient access challenges • Operational impediments • Fragmentation of oncology services • Communication challenges with oncologists and referring doctors • Oncology surgery referrals leaving the hospital and outpatient clinics	**Avoid** • Mentality of "defending turf" • Alienation of aligned community physicians • Exclusion of key stakeholders from decision-making process • Ambiguous governance and management structure • Poor patient outcomes

Source: ECG Management Consultants, Inc.

Strategic Planning for Oncology Services

After formulating a vision for the future of oncology and a goals grid, the next step is to develop explicit goals that identify the achievements the organization intends to accomplish. Typically, strategic goals relate to things such as financial performance, physician relations, and coordination of services. They highlight the specific areas of activity and should be measurable and time specific. Examples of oncology goals include the following:

- Five percent increase in inpatient oncology market share within 36 months

- Add two oncologists to the medical staff within 24 months

- Add two exclusive physician relationships for oncology within 12 months

- Attain National Comprehensive Cancer Control Program designation within 24 months

- Implement two value-based payment projects with health plans within 18 months

- Achieve a 15% increase in clinical research within 18 months

- Implement 10 patient care protocols within 18 months

- Achieve and maintain an average of 8.5 on patient satisfaction scores within 24 months

- Initiate two multidisciplinary oncology clinics within 24 months

- Develop two oncology clinics outside of the primary market area within 24 months

Chapter 1

Step 5: Making It Happen

A vision and set of goals address what the organization wants to do; tactics address how it will be done. Tactics are the specific initiatives and action steps that will be taken in order to achieve each goal. Tactics should include accountabilities and target dates for each specific action (Figure 1.5 examines the last goal from the list above and provides possible tactics).

FIGURE 1.5

SAMPLE GOAL: INITIATE TWO ONCOLOGY CLINICS OUTSIDE OF THE PRIMARY MARKET AREA WITHIN 24 MONTHS

	Tactic	Accountability	Due Date
1.	Collect and evaluate data from potential markets	Smith	1/15
2.	Select top four markets for further evaluation	Team	1/30
3.	Identify real estate, hospital relationship, and other operational issues for each potential site	Smith	2/30
4.	Prepare business plan for best two locations	Smith/Jones	3/30
5.	Secure steering committee and board approval	Smith	4/14
6.	Execute lease(s) and finalize operational timeline	Smith/Brown	5/1

Source: ECG Management Consultants, Inc.

If tactics are well defined for each goal as shown previously, the organization has a clear road map for achieving strategic goals. This is, in fact, the strategic plan for oncology. It is recommended that tactics be reviewed every six months for necessary changes, while a full review of progress on each goal area is made annually.

Often, most failed strategies result from failures of implementation, rather than a failure of the strategy itself. The cost of a failed strategy includes potential alienation of physician leadership, frustrated management, and wasted resources. In addition, the organization has given its competition an opportunity to take advantage of its lack of progress. Successful implementation of the plan is critically important and is dependent on the tactics, accountabilities, and timelines that the team has adopted. It is hard work to think through and document each tactical step for every goal within the vision, but this is the work that enables execution of the strategy. The importance of a tactical plan cannot be overestimated. In addition, engaging physicians in the implementation process is of paramount importance. The medical staff can be a key ally for implementing tactical actions to improve performance, enhance quality, and gain market share. If not, the medical staff may become a formidable obstacle along the pathway to change.

Learning from experience: Basic strategic themes

There are a number of ways to develop and evaluate strategies, and the right method is the one that encourages a thoughtful dialogue and seeks to ensure that the strategies will help the organization achieve its future vision. It is critical for the key stakeholders who are driving the strategic planning process to evaluate all potential strategies to ascertain their implications and ensure their fit. Specifically, the types of questions that should be asked include:

Chapter 1

- From a market perspective, which strategy will best allow us to grow market share and volumes?

- Operationally, will this strategy enable us to improve quality, service, and efficiency?

- Which scenario offers the best financial potential?

- Can we afford the investments in capital, physicians, and technology required to achieve this strategic scenario?

- Are there political barriers that will hinder us in achieving this scenario? Are they surmountable?

One of the biggest questions that leadership needs to agree on for any potential strategic plan is how "game changing" the strategies need to be. For example, does the organization need transformational or directional strategies? For a hospital that is facing grave issues with its medical staff or a sharp loss in volume, the answer is probably the former. Transformational strategies are ones that seek to be disruptive to the market in order to shift current trends. They create significant change, both internally and, if successful, in the market. Other organizations are not looking for a sea change, but instead need to refocus and refine existing efforts. This could mean reevaluating the technological needs of the program, reinvigorating outreach efforts, or adding clinical scope to the service. A directional strategy is still powerful, but it does not have the level of change or the level of risk inherent in a transformational strategy. Understanding key stakeholders' expectations for the strategic plan and the level of change that it will create is important

Strategic Planning for Oncology Services

because one of the keys to successful execution is making sure that the plan is supported by hospital leadership.

Most strategies revolve around several basic themes. In nearly all regions, the markets are mature, and there is limited growth in the potential size of the market. Thus, the growth is driven by capturing additional market share from competitors. To do this, most organizations create focused strategies to differentiate themselves from their competitors in the eyes of patients and physicians. This may mean a focus on technology and being on the cutting edge. Conversely, it could mean focusing on outreach in growing communities or directly targeting competitors' current strongholds. Other hospitals use facilities to differentiate themselves, focusing on creating an institute or cancer center that contains the continuum of oncology services and creates a physical presence in the community. What all these market capture strategies have in common is taking advantage of opportunities in the market and allocating the resources to make it possible.

Strategic themes

In order to further define the strategic direction, the collective results of analysis (qualitative and quantitative) can be developed into a strategic theme (see Figure 1.6). The theme can be used as an overarching framework for the development of the tactical and implementation planning. With oncology service line planning, there is a spectrum ranging from a virtual cancer center to a comprehensive cancer program, with an intermediary consolidated program. They are defined as the following:

Chapter 1

- Virtual cancer center: Incremental growth and coordination of existing oncology services provided by a hospital, oncology physician groups, and others.

- Consolidated program: Development of a more coordinated program in a medical office building facility that aggregates key physicians into a single location, increases physician leadership, and advances research efforts.

- Comprehensive cancer program: Development of a comprehensive program with tumor site focus, a hub of cancer care (a center) that houses all cancer treatment and support services, and a research alliance with a prominent program. The highest level of integration will be achieved through tight alignment with physicians, through employment, or through other models.

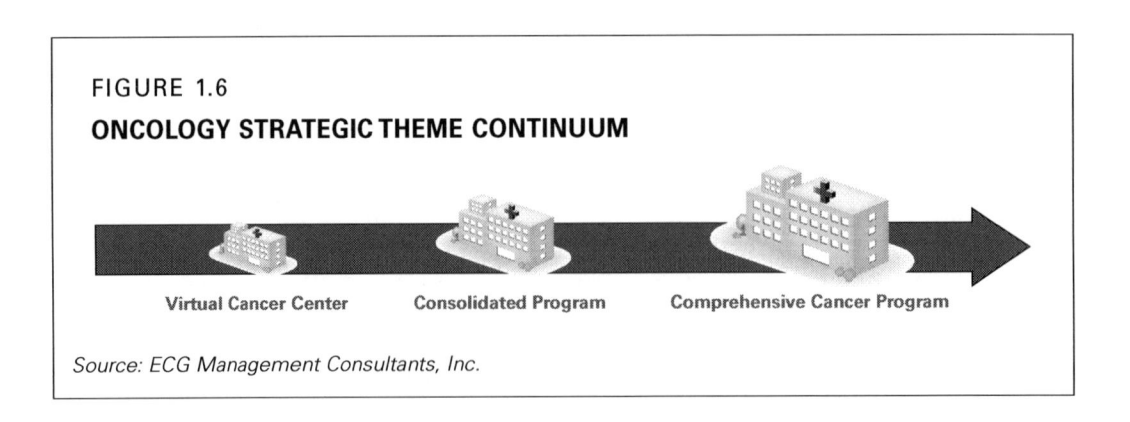

FIGURE 1.6
ONCOLOGY STRATEGIC THEME CONTINUUM

Virtual Cancer Center → Consolidated Program → Comprehensive Cancer Program

Source: ECG Management Consultants, Inc.

Typically, the model/theme selected is driven by the desired attributes of the clinical program and level of clinical integration/coordination. The remaining thematic elements are designed to support the desired characteristics. The strategic themes can be compared using eight key characteristics for cancer programs:

coordination, clinical programs, facilities, physician alignment, research, patient support services, institutional affiliation, and technology. Figure 1.7 is an example comparison of the strategic themes based on these key characteristics. The themes illustrated here are representative of the general progression/evolution of cancer programs; in reality, the themes outlined in the figure are infinitely flexible and can be adapted to any organization's unique circumstances.

FIGURE 1.7
ONCOLOGY STRATEGIC THEME

Characteristic	Virtual Cancer Center	Consolidated Program	Comprehensive Cancer Program
Coordination	• Expansion of current navigation services • Incremental development of tumor boards	• Expansion of current navigation services • Development of select tumor teams • Development of clinical pathways • Development of health information exchange for clinical information	• Expansion of current navigation services • Tumor-specific multi-disciplinary clinics • Physician-led organization • Integrated electronic medical record (EMR)
Clinical programs	• Clinical programs based on current tumor-site expertise and physician interest	• Clinical programs will be developed and expanded based on population and market trends	• Clinical programs developed and expanded based on population and market trends

Chapter 1

FIGURE 1.7
ONCOLOGY STRATEGIC THEME (CONT.)

Characteristic	Virtual Cancer Center	Consolidated Program	Comprehensive Cancer Program
Clinical programs (cont.)	• Incremental development of tumor boards	• Limited development of clinical protocols • Increasing multidisciplinary care (e.g., tumor boards and tumor teams); likely focused in one or two areas of clinical expertise	• Development of sub-specialty expertise • Recruitment of physicians with tumor-site expertise • Development of tumor teams and tumor-specific "institutes" • Focus on developing clinical protocols
Facilities	• Facility upgrades will be minimal and limited to existing centers	• Develop new facility with oncology therapy, diagnostic, and support services • Explore development of outpatient facilities in the community	• A new, state-of-the art, easily accessible cancer center would be constructed • The center would include radiation oncology • The facility would house therapy, diagnostic, and support services
Physician alignment	• Medical directorships	• Joint ownership of ancillaries	• Economic alignment of providers through a single organization

FIGURE 1.7
ONCOLOGY STRATEGIC THEME (CONT.)

Characteristic	Virtual Cancer Center	Consolidated Program	Comprehensive Cancer Program
Physician alignment (cont.)	• Physician-led programs	• Infusion therapy partnerships • Service line comanagement	• Participation in bundled payment or shared savings programs • Service line comanagement
Research	• Research focus is limited to continuing current research efforts	• Moderate growth in research focus • Improved patient access to research and clinical protocols through affiliation • Improved marketing of research efforts through cancer program • Potential expansion of research services to include surgery or radiation therapy	• Strong research focus • Improved patient access to research and clinical protocols • Affiliation with major cancer program • Recruitment of physicians with research interest • Investigator-initiated studies and/or expansion of research services to include surgery or radiation therapy
Patient support services	• Coordination and communication of current support services • Expansion of patient navigators	• Begin adding more support services (e.g., nutrition counseling) • Consolidate support services in one location • Market support services	• Full continuum of support services provided at the cancer center • Navigators coordinating care, especially in outlying clinics • Development of new services

Chapter 1

FIGURE 1.7

ONCOLOGY STRATEGIC THEME (CONT.)

Characteristic	Virtual Cancer Center	Consolidated Program	Comprehensive Cancer Program
Institutional affiliation	• Branding/marketing	• Branding/marketing • Research • Provider education	• Branding/marketing • Access to sub-specialists and/or quaternary care • Research • Clinical protocols • Provider education
Technology	• Nominal investment in technology • Expansion of communication capabilities	• Perhaps new, dedicated, diagnostic services (PET/CT, MRI) as joint ventures	• Fully integrated EMR • Investment in innovative imaging and diagnostic tools • Acquisition of leading-edge therapeutic technology

Source: ECG Management Consultants, Inc.

It is important to keep the vision and goals previously developed for the program in mind when reviewing the strategic themes, considering the benefits and challenges of each, and ultimately selecting one that aligns with the program. With each strategic theme, there are clinical, financial, operational, and political implications. On the comprehensive cancer program side of the spectrum, there is greater risk, but there is also potential for more benefits (clinical, financial, etc.). For example, the virtual cancer center would have minimal financial investment requirements, and program growth would likely be somewhat limited. In contrast, the comprehensive cancer program would initially require a significant capital investment.

Through the formation of a comprehensive cancer program, the service line would be better positioned to advance clinical care, increase clinical research, and improve patient volumes. In the end, the goal is to identify the most appropriate strategy for the organization, one that capitalizes on its strengths, minimizes its weaknesses, and propels the program toward its goals. Setting this foundation will be critical to selecting which tactics and initiatives to pursue.

Key Takeaways

At its heart, strategic planning is about resource allocation and determining the programs or initiatives that will be the focus of the hospital's resources. No cookbook exists to lay out the exact recipe for developing the optimal strategies. A good strategy is grounded in the past, which is the reason for the situational assessment, but looks to the future, which is why the vision is at the apex of the planning process. Goal development ensures that the hospital has a clear idea of what it wishes to accomplish, and carefully documented tactics ensure that it will, in fact, reach its goals.

The key points to keep in mind regarding strategic planning are:

- Involve key stakeholders in both the development and execution of the strategic plan

Chapter 1

- Be realistic in assessing both what the organization can accomplish in theory and what it is willing to commit in terms of resources

- Don't take shortcuts in the progression from vision to goals to strategies to tactics

- Understand that course corrections and plan revisions will be needed

CHAPTER 2

Creating a Successful Oncology Service Line

During the past several decades, extraordinary advances in oncology care have dramatically increased the likelihood of survival for cancer patients and promised an improved quality of life for survivors. Despite this progress, the market for oncology services continues to be characterized by inconsistent access to care, limited coordination among providers, frequent variability in treatment, and rapidly increasing costs. The passage of healthcare reform and a number of innovative payment mechanisms being introduced by both public and private payers (e.g., accountable care organizations, bundled payments, and pay for performance) have brought these issues to the forefront. In the future, successful oncology services will be characterized by the following:

- Delivering care that is coordinated across providers, specialties, and sites of service

- Offering high-quality diagnostic, therapeutic, and support services in a patient-centric setting

- Adhering to evidence-based oncology practice guidelines and eliminating unnecessary variability in treatment protocols

- Improving access to care and the coordination of services as the economics of healthcare delivery shift from volume to value

Chapter 2

In an effort to adapt to the evolving cancer delivery and payment model, many hospitals are developing oncology service line structures that improve performance, encourage physician involvement, and create a distinct brand in the market to ultimately gain competitive advantage. The level of activity varies widely among hospitals, but there is broad agreement that structuring oncology as a service line within the hospital or health system is necessary for success.

This chapter provides an introduction to service line principles and the areas that should be considered to ensure a successful oncology service line. Topics to be covered include the following:

- Introduction to service line principles

- Key elements for service line success

- Implementation issues

- The future for oncology service lines

Introduction to Service Line Principles

A service line is organized around patient diagnosis to provide coordination of care and accessibility of information over time, regardless of where the care is provided or who provides it. Service lines are typically recognizable to patients and caregivers as a conglomeration of inpatient and ambulatory services that a patient may require during treatment for an episode or condition. The service line management concept has been used since the early part of the twentieth century to coordinate resources and functions that respond to the market. Despite its wide-scale implementation across numerous industries, the approach was not widely utilized in healthcare until the mid- to late 1980s. Service lines have seen a renewed emphasis in recent years as hospitals look for ways to create an identified brand in the market and drive clinical and financial performance. Interest in service line structures has been accelerated by an increased emphasis on ambulatory care and acquisition of physician practices by hospitals. In many organizations, however, the concept is not well defined and is largely misunderstood.

For years, hospitals have advanced and/or marketed a range of programs under the heading "service line," and it is no surprise that the concept is now a bit unclear for most observers. Groupings of complementary services do not constitute a service line unless the following features are also present:

- Viewed by physicians, management, and patients as a coordinated array of services needed for specified conditions

- Provides a single point of patient access throughout the treatment process

- Offers coordinated provider teams for patient-based services and care

- Incorporates standardized processes, protocols, and outcome measurements

- Reports financial, operational, and quality-of-care data at the service line level

- Demands alignment of physicians, staff, and management across all sites of care

Chapter 2

- Offers participation in strategic, operational, and financial decision-making for key providers

- Operates under a unified control structure that governs critical operations and the strategy regarding service line delivery assets

Oncology and cardiovascular programs are the most common service lines within hospitals, followed by women and children, neuroscience, and orthopedics. Smaller and/or more narrowly focused programs can also meet the criteria for service line development and should be given consideration, especially if physician leadership is available.

Key Elements for Service Line Success

The key elements to consider in developing a new service line or enhancing an existing one are:

- Services provided

- Governance structure

- Management structure

- Physician alignment

- Financial structure

- Facilities

- Information technology

Services provided

The first and most basic question hospitals should ask themselves is: "What services are included?" Due to the program requirements of many cancer services, this question requires careful thought and input from clinicians. For example, Figure 2.1 portrays a typical list of oncology services that may be appropriate for a fully developed service line.

FIGURE 2.1

TYPICAL SERVICES INCLUDED IN A COMPREHENSIVE ONCOLOGY SERVICE LINE

Diagnostic	Therapeutic	Support Services	Research	Education and Outreach
• X-ray • Fluoroscopy • Ultrasound • CT • MRI • Nuclear medicine • PET/CT • Mammography • Endoscopy • Colonoscopy • Biopsy • Tumor marker • Lab	• Hematology/oncology • Infusion therapy • Radiation therapy • Surgical oncology • Gynecologic oncology • Plastic/reconstructive surgery • Multidisciplinary clinics	• Patient navigation • Rehabilitation • Pain and palliative care • Nutritional counseling • Mental health and social work • Financial counseling • Integrative medicine • Survivorship program	• Clinical research trials • Research physicians • Academic cancer program affiliation	• Cancer screenings • Community health fairs and seminars • Continuing medical education for physicians • Patient education materials and programs • Self-assessment risk questionnaires

Source: ECG Management Consultants, Inc.

Once an organization has determined which services to include in the service line, the organization must then determine how to enhance coordination amongst those services. Coordinating the delivery of services and making them accessible to

Chapter 2

patients as part of a multidisciplinary service line is complex, particularly given the fragmented nature of oncology care. In most markets, the majority of oncology business (i.e., infusion and radiation therapy) takes place in freestanding outpatient centers outside the confines of the hospital and is controlled by multiple, independent, and often competing business entities. Bringing this diverse group of players together to provide coordinated treatment and optimize patient care requires well-defined organization, governance, and management structures.

Organizational model

Service lines are emerging as the organizational backbone of many hospitals, with well-defined clinical and business units replacing the traditional siloed management structure. For example, the ultimate cancer service line organization model will span both outpatient and inpatient settings, allowing for a more coordinated approach to achieving strategic and operational objectives, as well as improving accountability throughout the organization for patient outcomes and service. The increased span of control, under either a prominent physician leader, senior executive, or both, is a result of the health system dedicating resources, political capital, and effort to its cancer strategy.

Some of the key decision-making authorities that generally vary with the service line model chosen are budgetary control and hiring/termination of staff and physicians within the service line. Organizations that grant the service line executive with real authority by giving him/her these critical management responsibilities can dramatically increase the effectiveness of the service line, regardless of structure. However, if an organization is seeking the most integrated model and does not provide the physician leadership structure with these responsibilities, it will substantially reduce the ability of management to achieve the desired results of the more highly integrated model.

When choosing a service line structure, an organization should understand the advantages and disadvantages of several models and understand how the unique characteristics of its existing leaders and services fit within each. While an administrator or nurse executive typically oversees oncology service line management, clinical integration is dependent upon the effectiveness of the physician leadership structure. The continuum of organizational structures is described in Figure 2.2, which provides a summary of the common governance options for oncology service lines.)

FIGURE 2.2
RANGE OF ONCOLOGY SERVICE LINE GOVERNANCE STRUCTURES

Type of Structure	Description	Relative Effort Required for Implementation	Relative Effectiveness
Matrixed	Key and shared services have a matrix/limited reporting relationship to a service line coordinator.	Medium	Low to medium
Partially consolidated	Key service line areas report directly to a senior-level service line director. Other areas have only an indirect (i.e., dotted line) reporting relationship.	Medium	Medium
Fully integrated	All areas within a service line report directly to a senior-level service line director, who is fully dedicated to overseeing operations and development.	High	High

Source: ECG Management Consultants, Inc.

Chapter 2

Matrixed structure

In a traditional organizational model, departments have separate reporting relationships with minimal or informal coordination and overlap of functional expertise. One way that organizations with a traditional model create a more integrated service line is by developing a matrixed reporting structure (see Figure 2.3). This model designates a position for a service line coordinator, who has limited or no direct responsibilities for the departments that compose the service line. Instead, he or she has relationships with the directors and managers of the key departments and acts in an advisory role, rather than offering direct oversight.

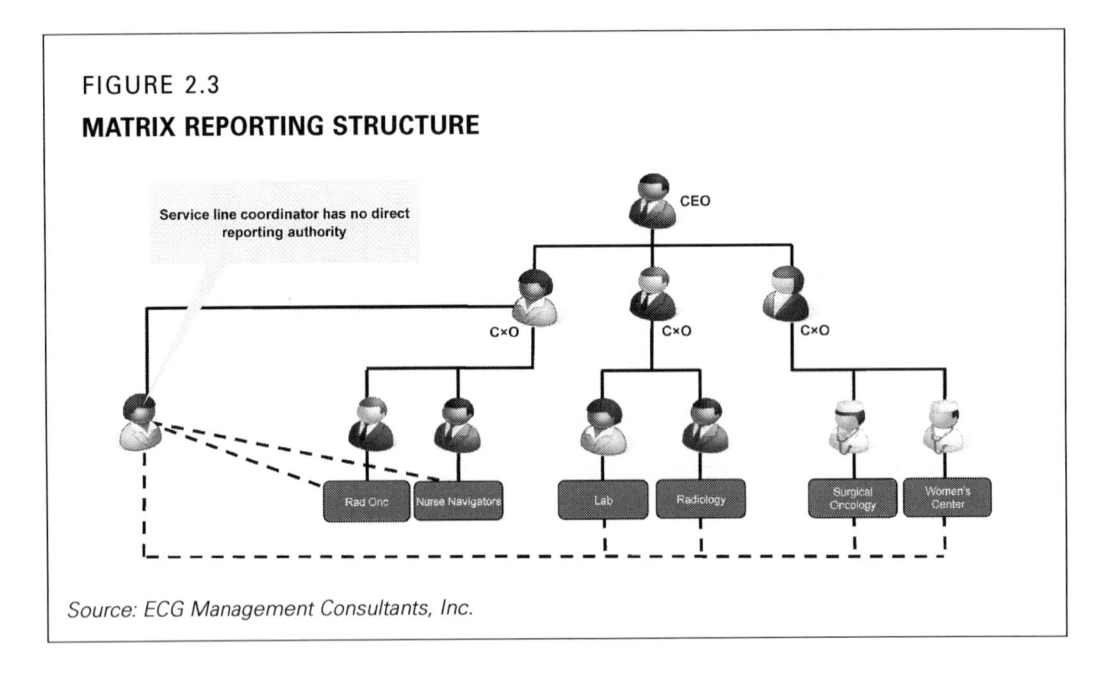

FIGURE 2.3
MATRIX REPORTING STRUCTURE

Service line coordinator has no direct reporting authority

Source: ECG Management Consultants, Inc.

While this model begins to create a service line focus, the coordinator is operating in an environment in which he or she is facilitating efforts but has no direct control. The individual usually has a business and physician development skill set and

38 © 2011 HealthLeaders Media — Oncology: Strategies for Superior Service Line Performance

works to guide new program development. The trade-off with not centralizing direct oversight is that this structure can cause delays in the decision-making process because multiple parties need to be consulted before key decisions are made. Further, the success of these matrix reporting structures is greatly dependent upon the individuals in the various roles working well together.

Partially consolidated structure

In a partially consolidated structure, depicted in Figure 2.4, a service line administrator has direct responsibility for some, but not all, key departments. He or she has a matrix relationship with those departments that do not fall under the purview of the service line. For example, the cancer service line director will nearly always have control over support services (e.g., nutrition, social work) and hospital-based infusion and radiation therapy. More difficult to determine are the reporting relationships for inpatient, surgical, and imaging services, which may have an indirect reporting relationship to the cancer service line director. Such frameworks are common when political barriers prevent changes to the control structure for key departments or services. A partially consolidated structure can work efficiently, particularly if most key departments are centralized under service line management and there are strong working relationships with other key directors and managers. As with any matrix structure, it is critical to specifically define what is signified by the dotted line.

Chapter 2

FIGURE 2.4

PARTIALLY CONSOLIDATED REPORTING STRUCTURE

Source: ECG Management Consultants, Inc.

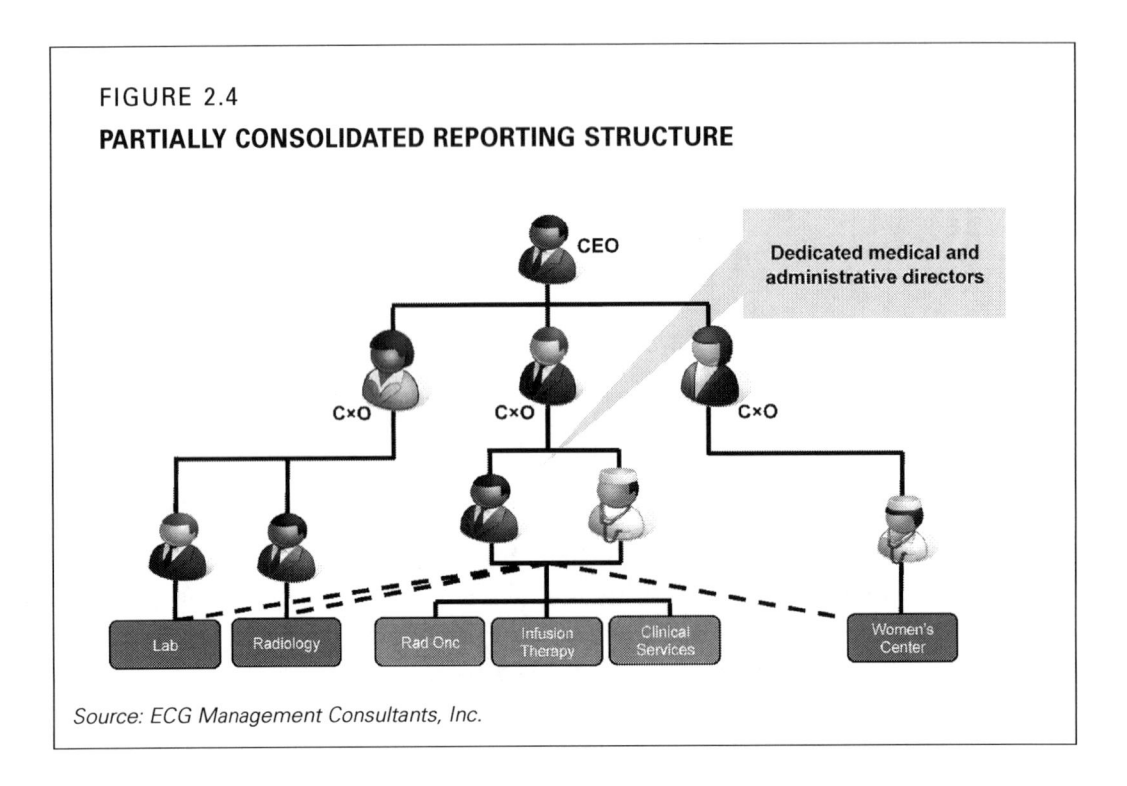

Fully integrated structure

Under a fully integrated model (Figure 2.5), the health system views the service line as the primary organizational unit. Ideally, functional areas/departments (nursing, information technology, finance, etc.) will view the oncology service line director as an important client, and he/she will report directly to the chief operating officer or CEO, as shown in the figure. Like the other structures, this model has trade-offs, specifically that decisions can sometimes be made in a vacuum without fully considering the impact on non-oncology departments. However, physicians and managers tend to function well in this structure, because it simplifies the decision-making process.

Creating a Successful Oncology Service Line

FIGURE 2.5
FULLY INTEGRATED REPORTING STRUCTURE

Dedicated oversight for service line; all service line-related services report to dyad management team

Source: ECG Management Consultants, Inc.

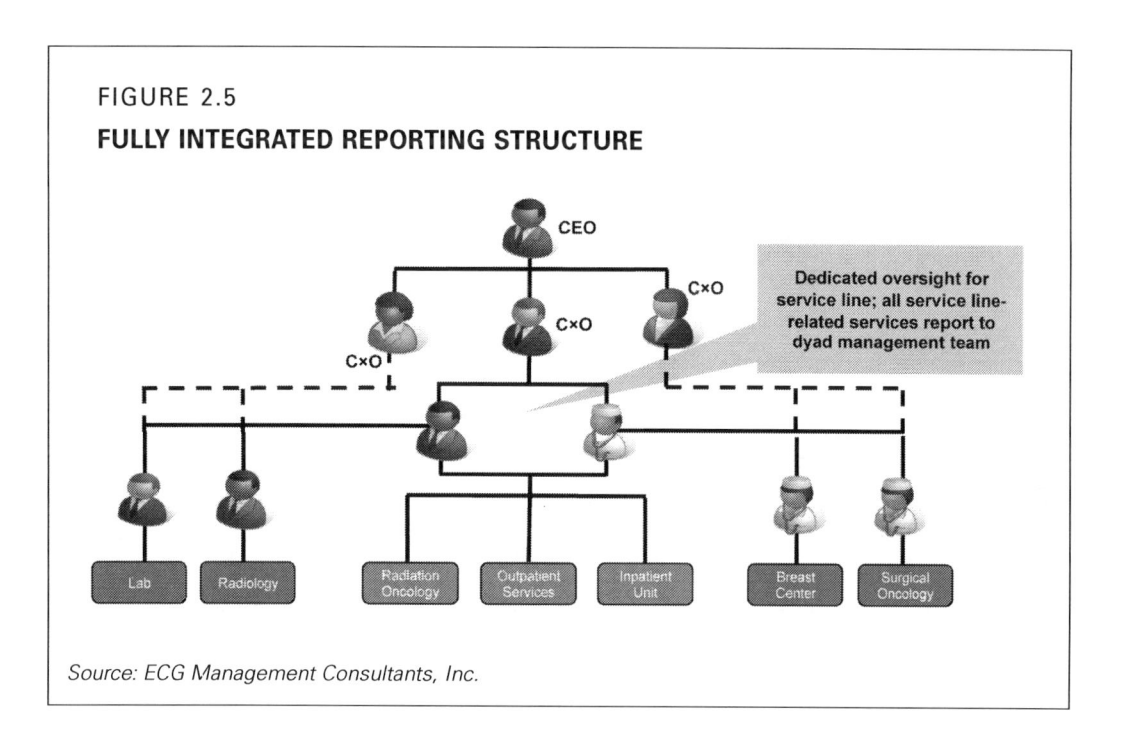

Regardless of the organizational construct in place, many elements critical to the success of the service line will likely exist outside the institutional control of the organization. A typical market may have infusion services provided predominantly in freestanding centers owned and operated by one or more private practice medical oncology or multispecialty oncology groups. Radiation oncology services may be furnished by a separate group or multiple groups that own their own linear accelerators (LINAC), increasingly in conjunction with large for-profit firms that operate radiation therapy centers nationally, or staff a hospital-owned LINAC. Surgeons and other specialists involved in oncology care may belong to separate physician groups and be affiliated with the hospital independently. It is obviously important for the service line management team to work collaboratively with

Chapter 2

independent physicians, medical groups, and other providers or oncology services. A responsive governance structure with appropriate physician representation and involvement is equally important.

Systemwide service lines

Creating an oncology service line that spans multiple hospitals in a health system presents both an opportunity and a challenge. The ability to work as a coordinated entity to manage resources and route patients within the system to the appropriate facility for care represents a tremendous opportunity for the growth of services, enhanced coordination of care, and expense management. Consolidating services and even constructing a dedicated cancer center offer advantages to elevate market differentiation and attract both patients and providers to the facility. However, operational and political considerations make this challenging. Given that many cancer care providers, such as surgeons, are not exclusive to oncology patients, it is sometimes politically and operationally difficult to consolidate these services. The degree of systemness currently in place magnifies this challenge. In fragmented systems of care, where each hospital operates in relative isolation, the challenge of creating coordination between hospitals will be difficult to overcome. If the hospitals have a precedent for allocating resources at a system level, these issues can be more easily resolved.

The overall goal of implementing a service line at the system level is to enhance the value to patients, resulting in market share gains. The management and governance structures are what allow this level of coordination to take place. In the case of a system, this may mean providing diagnostic testing and infusion therapy services at the local level and then routing the patients to the tertiary care facility for subspecialized care and surgical intervention. Many of the same principles previously discussed apply, but they involve participants from each hospital. For management, this may mean creating a system level cancer services management position to ensure appropriate coordination, standardization, and allocation of resources at all facilities.

A key question that must be answered is: To what extent should the services be actively managed at a system level, versus by hospital site? In most cases, it makes sense to manage day-to-day operations at the hospital level, with high-level coordination provided by the system. Distances between hospitals and the level of services offered at each impact these choices. In terms of governance, participants from all hospitals must be involved. The governance committee then often reports to the system CEO or a designated executive charged with leading the service line. Within a system, only the people involved and the individuals to whom the governing board reports change; the goals for the governance structure remain the same. System versus local and/or regional authorities and responsibilities will need careful consideration and are highly dependent on market and clinical factors.

Physician alignment

Achieving physician alignment is perhaps the single most important factor in the development of a successful service line. At the same time, it is often the most difficult element of the oncology service line to achieve, given the relationships between hospitals and oncology-related physicians as they have traditionally existed in most markets.

Chapter 2

The critical objectives of most oncology programs—growth; integrated, multidisciplinary care; consistent patient care protocols and outcome measures; enhanced patient experiences; and meaningful efficiency improvements—simply are not likely to emerge if traditional relationships are maintained. The basic alternatives for a hospital range from offering medical directorships (essentially buying clinical input), to developing contractual relationships (comanagement, lease arrangements, joint ventures, gain sharing, etc.), or to employing physicians. There are benefits and drawbacks to each of the options. However, our experience suggests that a combination of approaches may be most useful and practical, depending on the unique characteristics of each situation.

In addition to the relationship between physicians and the hospital, consideration must be given to the relationships among different oncology specialties that will be part of the service line. The interdisciplinary nature of oncology services places a premium on cooperation between physicians. Promoting collaboration, especially among physicians who may be competing for patients or resources, is a major management challenge. Figure 2.6 depicts some of the structural variety in these relationships and the implications of each.

Creating a Successful Oncology Service Line

FIGURE 2.6
PHYSICIAN ALIGNMENT CONSTRUCTS

State of Alignment	Description	Strategic Priorities
Competition	Each subspecialist is independently affiliated with the hospital. Clinical integration is lacking, and groups compete for patients and available resources.	• Forming a strong, physician-led governance body. • Building trust and coordination between groups through modest joint initiatives (e.g., service line dashboards, joint outreach clinics, coordinated physician referrals).
Coordination	Subspecialists remain independent but take a coordinated approach to referral relationships and physician recruitment.	• Clearly aligning economic incentives. • Creating more complex joint service line initiatives, such as program development and service line marketing.
Combination	Some specialists remain independent, while others are formally employed by the hospital.	• Building trust between employed and independent physicians. • Aligning the financial incentives of all physicians, regardless of employment status.
Coalition	All subspecialists are employed, resulting in a unified and coordinated physician workforce. Program planning, resource allocation, and physician recruitment are aligned.	• Developing a compensation plan that aligns physician and service line incentives and accounts for the unique needs of each individual subspecialty. • Ensuring physician engagement in service line planning and governance.

Source: ECG Management Consultants, Inc.

Financial structure

The familiar hospital financial management systems, characterized by granular cost centers and more general revenue reports, are not well suited to the cross-divisional and multidisciplinary management needs of most service lines. To accurately measure financial performance, each service line should be accounted for as if it is a separate business unit, with all revenue and all costs allocated back to the service line. For example, if a patient with breast cancer is seen in the clinic, has a biopsy performed, then has a surgical procedure followed by a hospital stay, all revenue from all three services should be credited to the oncology service line. Likewise, the cost associated with each service should be charged to the service line through a system of transfer pricing within the hospital. The task of allocating revenues and expenses to a particular service line takes on added complexity in

Chapter 2

instances where individuals suffer from multiple diagnoses and comorbidities, as is often the case for oncology patients (see Figure 2.7 for a range of financial reporting structures). While difficult to achieve, basing accounting on service lines can provide significantly improved data for the management of the organization, ultimately enabling better decisions on resource allocation.

FIGURE 2.7
RANGE OF FINANCIAL REPORTING STRUCTURES

Model	Description	Considerations	Relative Effort and Effectiveness
Traditional reporting	Traditional structure; each cost department is accountable for creating and maintaining its own budget (e.g., infusion, lab, imaging, and operating room all have separate budgets and financial statements).	Requires no additional implementation. Necessitates a manual collection process. Provides ambiguous reports on overall service line performance because of different reporting systems.	Low
Structured service line reporting	Partially integrated financial structure; some financial reporting methods are consolidated to provide more comprehensive service line performance reports.	Requires the development of a standardized reporting process to ensure the development of comparable financial reports. Provides some indication of overall performance, but results are often still ambiguous. Is a somewhat labor-intensive process.	Medium (depending on extent of decision support services)
Integrated service line reporting	Fully integrated financial structure; the oncology service line has one budget for all oncology-related facility and management services and reports integrated financial statements.	Offers the most accurate method for assessing service line performance. Requires a more comprehensive financial reporting system. May be a labor- and cost-intensive implementation process.	High (depending on extent of decision support services)

Source: ECG Management Consultants, Inc.

Facilities

From an oncology patient's perspective, being able to see all major components of the continuum of care immediately upon entering the lobby can have important psychological and physical benefits. Having services located in close proximity not only reduces the time, energy, and anxiety associated with scheduling and travel to multiple appointments, but gives patients and their families the feeling that care is being provided in a unified manner. Colocating related services also helps to foster specialist interactions and facilitate multidisciplinary care by allowing a team of providers from various disciplines to evaluate patients and develop a treatment plan that incorporates multiple perspectives. From a practical standpoint, colocation can help reduce travel time for staff and allow for more immediate identification of work flow and bottleneck issues.

Freestanding cancer centers are the ultimate goal of most oncology programs, but they are difficult to achieve because of the capital required, as well as potential inefficiencies of duplicating existing hospital services at a new site.

The most significant obstacles for an oncology service line will likely be bringing together providers from different specialties and groups and integrating clinic activity with hospital-based services. Nevertheless, a facility strategy needs to be part of any service line plan. At a minimum, a hospital should group service line components as close together as is practical. Other details, such as a dedicated entry and common signage, will provide comfort to patients, impart a sense of coordination, and help establish a brand identity. The continuum of facility options is illustrated in Figure 2.8.

Chapter 2

FIGURE 2.8
RANGE OF FACILITY OPTIONS

Typical Progression

Clinical Program
- Shared medical and surgical facilities, with limited dedicated procedure areas or ORs.
- No subspecialty patient clinics.
- Diagnostic ancillaries available but are a shared resource.
- All administration and marketing take place at the hospitalwide level.

Service Line
- Dedicated entry/lobby area with external signage.
- Range of integrated subspecialty services, with a multidisciplinary approach to service line patients (e.g., medical, surgical, radiation oncology).
- Highly focused on one or two therapeutic modalities.
- Multidisciplinary clinics and case review.
- Important services located in proximity to each other, but some services are scattered.

Institute Model
- Designated facility, typically freestanding or "hospital within a hospital."
- Facility would house comprehensive range of surgical and medical services offered, with emphasis on treatment of complex disorders.
- Tightly integrated with key specialties in other disciplines (e.g., urology).
- Generally associated with a research organization or academic department.
- Often a distinct brand from sponsoring hospital.

Source: ECG Management Consultants, Inc.

Information technology

In an oncology service line, the primary objective of any information technology (IT) deployed should be to enhance multidisciplinary care coordination and inform decision-making by care providers. Accordingly, the IT strategy should focus on the selection and implementation of an effective electronic medical record (EMR) and development of health information exchanges that facilitate the flow of clinical information among providers.

Key functional elements for an oncology EMR include the following:

- Drug sequencing and administration

- Support for tumor staging

- Toxicology monitoring

- Drug inventory management

- Data exchange from multiple databases (e.g., laboratory, radiology, pathology)

- Automated pharmacy ordering

- Patient support and communication

- Efficient revenue cycle processes

An effective EMR can also aid in charge capture and support the collection and reporting of data that is critical for measuring service line performance, including:

- Patient encounters by site

- Diagnosis

- Treatments

- Outcomes of care

Chapter 2

- Cost of care by diagnosis and treatment

- Financial performance of the service line

For most hospitals, EMRs are selected to meet the broad needs of multiple medical and surgical specialties. As such, existing systems are not likely to have the functionality required to support the complexities of oncology practice and will require modification to perform the elements described previously. This is typically accomplished through the addition of an oncology-specific module capable of interfacing with the general hospital EMR. Once selected, hospitals may wish to encourage adoption of the EMR by community physicians. This can be accomplished through a variety of strategies (e.g., financial subsidy, assistance with vendor selection, technical support) and serves not only to increase care coordination and efficiency, but can also help from a strategic standpoint to more closely align physicians with the hospital. Although IT decisions will be dictated by individual circumstances, oncology programs willing to invest the necessary staffing and information resources required will reap the benefits of improved patient care and service line performance.

Implementation Issues

Although designing the service line may present a variety of challenges to the organization, equally important, and perhaps more challenging, are implementation barriers. Typically, there are two major potential roadblocks to service line implementation: physician leadership and institutional culture. Chapter 3 explores, in greater detail, the role of physicians in providing program leadership and participating in governance activities of the service line.

Physician leadership

Oncology service line development demands tight alignment of physician and hospital interests, and getting there is often the most challenging aspect of service line management. Regardless of the structures used to align with physicians, hospitals with successful service lines acknowledge the requirement of physician champions and the importance of ceding true clinical and operational power to physician leaders. Physicians, for their part, often do not realize that the input they have long sought can be achieved through service line management. Nevertheless, few hospitals have ongoing programs to identify/develop physician leaders, and many of our clients find it frustrating to cultivate signature programs, because physician leadership cannot be found. From a different perspective, many of our academic health system clients have built distinguished clinical service lines due in large part to the power and visions of clinical department chairs.

Unfortunately, it is rare for a community hospital to have a physician with both the interest and the ability to lead a service line. It is frequently tempting to appoint the physician with the strongest technical skills to this position, the assumption being that the physician's strong clinical reputation corresponds with his or her ability to lead. However, the skills required more often resemble those of a compromise-crafting politician. Often, the hospital has to identify a physician with potential and then work to create the interest and skills necessary to be an effective leader. Hiring from the outside should be carefully thought out, because there is a danger of antagonizing existing providers. The challenge for CEOs is to first acknowledge the importance of physician leadership and then invest in the structure needed for it to happen.

Chapter 2

Institutional culture

Service lines demand the integration of traditionally siloed hospital functions. While this is a positive development for the reasons outlined previously, it represents a potentially significant change within the established hospital hierarchy. Management in nursing, finance, ancillary services, and employed physician clinics will be challenged to respond to service lines' needs in these environments. For instance, nursing within a service line may entail staffing for physician offices, diagnostic and procedure centers, patient education programs, and inpatient care. Oncology service line leadership will seek nurses with specific expertise who are dedicated to that service line and accountable to service line management. This may mean different pay levels for nurses, resistance to "floating" service line nurses to another unit, and a claim of ownership of the nursing staff by the service line. Nursing administration may have legitimate concerns related to education and enforcement of nursing standards and may resist accommodating such changes. Other hospital departments and members of the medical staff will face similar pressures, and intramural disputes can be expected. For hospital executives, the technical challenge of how best to organize an oncology service line may end up seeming easy compared to the management challenge of getting employees to embrace it.

The Future for Oncology Service Lines

It is appropriate to ask whether service lines are simply the most recent organizational fad or if they will have a longer-term impact on hospitals. In the near term, it is likely that hospitals will be focusing on the one, two, or three service lines that can best attract patients, providers, and payer contracts. For many—if not most—hospitals and health systems, this will include the oncology program. In this short-term scenario, service lines are essentially an add-on to the organization's business. Over time, however, service lines have the potential to be the organization's central business. Today's generalist hospital with limited coordination between hospital and ambulatory services will be replaced by coordinated groupings of inpatient and outpatient facilities interconnected by a shared organizational culture, value-driven leadership, and IT infrastructure. In most of today's tertiary centers and advanced community hospitals, an advanced oncology service line will be a critical component of that structure.

Fundamentally, service line development must be viewed as a major organizational commitment and should be carefully nurtured over time. It is likely that the future of an organization's service lines will determine the future of the organization as a whole. Because many organizations have begun this transformational process with their oncology programs, it may well be that this critical service sets the tone for the future of the organization and plays a critical role in its ability to compete in a rapidly changing healthcare marketplace.

Key Takeaways

Service lines should address each of the elements outlined previously; however, success is dependent on effective physician leadership. Coordinating care across many sites and specialties requires strong physician involvement and broadly based physician acceptance of the strategic aims under a cancer service line.

Chapter 2

Consideration, therefore, should been given to the following areas when developing an oncology service line plan:

- Engage physicians early in the planning process

- Identify key physician leaders/champions who can help create the vision and drive acceptance

- Carefully manage the breadth of views that are formally represented in the planning process to avoid getting mired down in politics

- Develop formal mechanisms (e.g. physician governance and physician alignment models) to support ongoing physician engagement with the program

- Provide physician leadership with regular updates on implementation progress

CHAPTER 3

The Importance of Governance and Leadership

The previous chapter detailed the key structural options and organizational elements for oncology service lines. It is equally important, and often more challenging, however, to create an environment for responsible policy setting and program oversight (governance), provide effective decision-making, and ensure efficient operations on a day-to-day basis (leadership). The critical element for successful governance and leadership is the incorporation of physicians in all aspects of designing, operating, evaluating, and enhancing oncology services. This chapter will discuss ways to structure governance and organize management to provide significant authority and accountability for physicians and facilitate the success of the oncology service line.

Oncology Governance Structures

An oncology service line can function with most policy settings and operations conducted by traditional hospital management structures or it can fully integrate physicians into both governance and leadership roles. Figure 3.1 illustrates increasing levels of physician involvement across the range of options.

Chapter 3

FIGURE 3.1
RANGE OF ONCOLOGY SERVICE LINE GOVERNANCE STRUCTURES

	Limited Governance	Ad Hoc Committee	Standing Committee	Governance Council
Overview	No established mechanism for governance. Individuals informally consulted.	Formed to discuss specific issues (e.g., new products, workforce planning) as they arise.	Established governance body responsible for wide range of oversight functions.	Board maintains complete accountability for service line performance, reporting directly to hospital CEO.
Strategic Planning	No role.	Informed.	Advisory.	Advice, direction, and approval.
Management Selection	No role.	Input into hiring.	Input into hiring, performance review.	Accountability for hiring and firing.
Budgeting	No role.	Occasional advisory.	Advisory.	Recommend.
Physician Composition	Individual physicians may be consulted.	Limited physician involvement.	Significant physician composition.	Majority physician composition.
Quality Monitoring	Can have separate CoC committee with emphasis on hospital services.	Separate CoC committee with little overlap to strategic and business operations.	Separate CoC Committee; quality measures tracked.	Quality reporting via subcommittee structure and CoC committee.

Increasing Degree of Complexity ➔

Source: ECG Management Consultants, Inc.

Although many oncology service lines function with minimal physician direction or leadership, the complexities of service line management and the difficulties of breaking down barriers between multiple care disciplines demand a high level of physician involvement. The governance structure should provide a forum for physicians and administration to come together to set the strategic direction for the service line and ensure that performance expectations are attained. Ideally, the governing body is an inclusive structure, composed of a select group of physicians

The Importance of Governance and Leadership

and senior executives from various clinical disciplines (e.g., surgical, medical, and radiation oncology). A service line governance structure that engages physicians will not only result in better decision-making and resource allocation but will also secure physician commitment to the service line's success. In short, any oncology service line that seeks to perform above minimal levels should include extensive physician participation in the functions of governance.

When developing a service line governance structure, it is necessary to consider how representation will be determined—specifically, the number of seats and how they might be apportioned across groups, specialties, or campuses. This is especially critical for oncology services because of the diverse array of providers involved and the potential for conflict across specialties and departments. Appointing a varied set of physician stakeholders helps to break down barriers between clinical areas.

> **WHAT ABOUT THE COC COMMITTEE?**
>
> It is useful to clarify the difference between the cancer committee specified by the American College of Surgeons Commission on Cancer (CoC) and the governance options in Figure 3.1. CoC accreditation includes appointing a multidisciplinary cancer committee to lead the program by setting goals, monitoring program activity, evaluating patient outcomes, and improving care.[1] It can be an important forum for quality assurance and oversight but typically does not provide the appropriate mechanism for strategic planning, business development, and operations improvement activities.

The responsibilities of a fully functioning governance structure include capital budgeting, facility planning, business development efforts, and maintaining accountability for service line performance. Typically, the governance body reports

Chapter 3

to the hospital CEO or another senior executive; this demonstrates the importance of this group and its role within the organization. However, it is important to note that this structure does not represent a corporate governance body with fiduciary authority. Service line governance is generally subordinate to the CEO and hospital board, but it provides an important forum for joint strategic planning and collaborative decision-making. As noted previously, it is crucial that the governance responsibilities are clear and relative to other existing administrative meetings, such as the hospital's cancer committee, because the governance group plays a pivotal role in the service line development and strategy and should limit participation to senior leaders who can elevate the discussion to key strategic and operational decisions.

Developing joint executive-physician governance is effective in demonstrating physicians' roles in the service line and the hospital's commitment to actively involving them in the program. It also provides physicians with a strong voice and a sense of decision-making authority in effecting change in the service line, as well as overall guidance to the future direction of the cancer program. A review of top-performing oncology service lines points to the formation of governance structures, such as a governance council, as critical to advancing the service line functions. The remainder of this section describes key elements of this construct.

Governance council membership

Membership of the service line governance council should be inclusive and represent all key constituents without becoming so large that decision-making is cumbersome (Figure 3.2). Typically, such a group has approximately 10 to 15 members, depending on services, physician makeup, and the number of facilities included in the service line. When the group size exceeds this size, it can be difficult to reach decisions, schedule meetings, and efficiently provide the required guidance for the program.

FIGURE 3.2
GOVERNANCE COUNCIL MEMBERSHIP

Executive Leadership	Physician Leadership
Oncology service line administrator	Medical director, oncology service line, chair
Chief financial officer or designee	Medical director, oncology
Chief nursing officer or designee	Medical director, oncological surgery
Chief operating officer or designee	Medical director, breast imaging center
Vice president, strategy and business development	Medical director, pathology
	Medical director, radiation oncology
	Medical director, clinical research (if applicable)
	Medical director, palliative care

Source: ECG Management Consultants, Inc.

The physicians appointed to this group will vary based on the structures at each hospital or system, as well as the number of physician groups practicing at the facility and the specialties included in the service line. If some of the physicians within the service line are employed, it is important that both employed and private practice physicians are included. This ensures that the group is representative, but, more importantly, it promotes alignment with the private physicians by seeking their support for the service line strategies. Often, a member of each key physician group is represented on the council to promote communication and give all constituents a voice in the service line. If there are employed practices, it is

Chapter 3

important to have strong links between the service line and the employed physician enterprise.

Ad hoc participants at governance council meetings can be invited to provide their perspectives and expertise on critical decisions. Examples of potential ad hoc members include the following:

- Other physicians, such as hospitalists, medical specialists associated with specific tumor programs, or primary care physicians

- Marketing representatives

- Physician liaisons

- Other nursing representatives

- Pharmacy directors

- Tumor registry representatives

- Department managers

- Business development representatives

- Facilities planning representatives

- Supply chain or purchasing managers

- Information technology representatives

ROLES AND RESPONSIBILITIES

Giving the governance council power is key to making the structure effective. The roles and responsibilities of the council vary depending on the level of control given to the group, but optimally, they include the following functions:

- Act as the governing body of the oncology service line, establishing the overall direction, and developing administrative policies and guidelines
- Establish the oncology service line's strategy and supporting business plan by:
    - Setting and prioritizing strategies for the service line
    - Developing administrative policies and guidelines
    - Overseeing business planning and operational activities
    - Overseeing physician recruitment activities
    - Directing supporting committees
    - Reviewing planning/implementation progress
    - Directing business development activities
- Oversee the budgeting process by:
    - Working collaboratively with service line administration to develop the budget
    - Prioritizing major capital expenditures
    - Providing input on key budget assumptions
- Maintain accountability for service line performance, including:
    - Monitoring outcomes metrics
    - Facilitating operating and capital budgeting
    - Reviewing adoption of new technology/procedures
    - Overseeing quality programs
    - Overseeing clinical research programs
    - Monitoring development of supportive care programs

Typically, the governance council reports to the CEO or, in certain cases, directly to the board of directors. Special consideration should be given to the role of the council in the budgeting process. This concept gives many CEOs pause because it seems to represent a fundamental change to the budgeting paradigm; however, established policies and procedures are not being replaced. Instead, the council will be asked to participate in the development of a budget for CEO approval. The budget process tends to be sufficiently balanced as there are typically one or more senior executives from the hospital participating in the governance council who can help to manage the expectations of the clinicians serving on the council. The council then must make difficult resource allocation choices and manage accordingly. Without at least this degree of authority over the budget, the governance council cannot have the level of control and authority needed to execute on service line strategies, and physicians are likely to view it as simply an advisory committee to management.

Potential subcommittee structures

Subcommittees are often used as work groups of the main governance council and are charged with addressing key areas of focus within the service line. The number of subcommittees should be limited to the most pressing and/or complex issues facing the organization. Typically, subcommittees include quality/outcomes, finance/operations, business development/outreach, and research/teaching. As specific strategic initiatives are pursued, the council may appoint ad hoc subcommittees or work groups to direct activities. These are frequently used when organizations are making specific investments in select tumor site programs and seek to engage a broad set of key stakeholders to drive planning and implementation.

Over time, the focus of the subcommittees can change to meet the needs of the service line.

The subcommittees should be viewed as the bodies charged with implementing and executing key strategies related to their area of focus, which should always be coordinated with the governance council. For instance, the strategic plan may include an initiative for coordination of care throughout the service line. The quality/outcomes management subcommittee would then be charged by the governance committee to execute on this strategy and provide routine reports to the council. In other settings, the quality/outcomes subcommittee would act as the CoC committee and bear responsibility for monitoring quality performance improvement initiatives. Members of the subcommittee would meet; create a plan for exploring key tactics, such as building a dashboard of metrics, creating standardized order sets, and utilizing patient navigators; and then report their continuing progress to the governing council.

These subcommittees can also be used as a tool for communication, as well as to bring new issues to the attention of the governance council. Subcommittee membership should not be limited to council members but should include a committee member acting as chair. Other physicians and administrative leaders should be involved, depending on the committee's area of focus. This creates broader involvement in governance and provides a means to disseminate information and to ensure that problems can progress through the system. For instance, the medical director for radiation oncology could advise the quality/outcomes subcommittee of an issue with nurses not appropriately communicating treatment instructions to patients. This would then be addressed in the subcommittee meeting, and the service line administrator and chief nursing officer would take appropriate action. Further, this might point to an issue in the overall training of staff and nurses, which could then be addressed by the governance council.

The key agenda items for the governance council should include standing meeting agenda items and critical strategic issues. Standing meeting agenda items to be presented at each meeting include a review of a dashboard of key metrics, reports from each subcommittee, and follow-up on questions from the last meeting. The bulk of the meeting should be devoted to discussing, providing input on, and reviewing key strategic initiatives. The initiatives to be discussed should flow from the annual strategic plan.

SAMPLE MEETING AGENDAS

The following sample meeting agendas illustrate how the governance council and subcommittees typically function.

Governance council:

- Review high-level performance dashboard

- Hear report from business development/outreach subcommittee on strengths and weaknesses of potential opportunities, and prioritize new outreach sites

- Charge business development/outreach subcommittee with designing business plan for next new site

- Discuss upcoming budget cycle and brainstorm potential capital needs

- Charge finance/operations subcommittee and administrator with composing first draft of budget

Quality/outcomes subcommittee:

- Determine key metrics to be monitored and presented at meetings

- Discuss additional technology or infrastructure needs to track metrics

- Review patient satisfaction data, and discuss key initiatives needed to target specific areas of improvement

- Discuss needs to market key outcomes metrics, and charge select committee members with researching best practices at other programs

Chapter 3

SAMPLE MEETING AGENDAS (CONT.)

Business development/outreach subcommittee:

- Review performance of current outreach sites

- Discuss and prioritize areas for improvement at current clinic sites

- Prioritize three or four potential outreach sites to be explored further

- Charge select committee members and administrator with performing evaluation of potential outreach opportunities

- Discuss physician and staff recruitment needs to staff outreach sites, and develop recommendations

Finance/operations subcommittee:

- Review key metrics indicative of service line performance

- Discuss highest-priority operational issues

- Charge administrator or designee in developing draft recommendation to address specific operational concerns

- Discuss upcoming budget cycle, and hear presentation describing the budgetary process

- Determine how finance/operations subcommittee can best interface in developing budget

Oncology Service Line Leadership

The question of day-to-day management and accountability for the performance of the oncology service line is often given too little thought. Consistent with most hospital management structures, operational leadership of the service line is commonly given to an administrator—usually an individual with direct management experience in one or more cancer-related departments. While such management is familiar and easy to implement, the interdisciplinary nature of service lines and the focus on physician alignment to drive clinical improvements require a physician-directed or shared management (dyad) model. Each model has its advantages and disadvantages, and there is no one-size-fits-all structure. Alternative approaches to leadership composition are shown in Figure 3.3.

Administrator-directed model

The administrator-led structure, which has been the most frequently used model, features a service line leader who understands the organizational, operational, and financial implications of running a cancer service line from a business standpoint. The challenge for the administrator is creating relationships with the various physicians and effecting change in areas such as clinical coordination, quality review and protocol development, standardization of supplies and equipment, and responsiveness to patient needs. These subjects can be successfully addressed only with physician leadership.

In organizations with a strong nursing culture, the administrator may be a nurse executive. The benefit of the nurse-led model is that the service line leader has a strong clinical focus and can maintain the nurse-to-nurse reporting relationships.

Chapter 3

FIGURE 3.3
APPROACHES TO ONCOLOGY SERVICE LINE LEADERSHIP

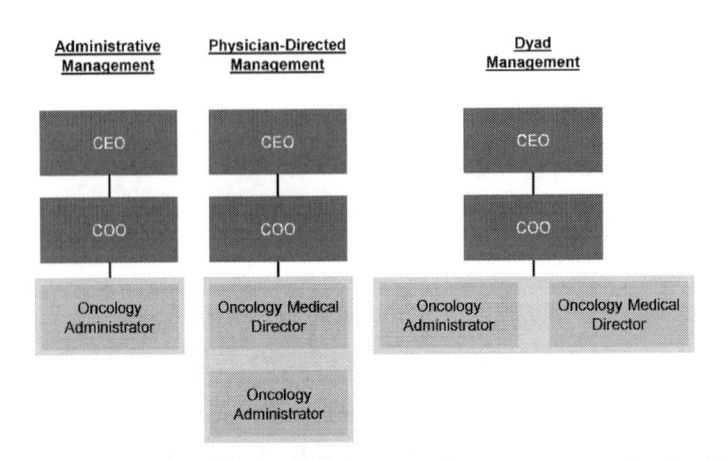

Administrative Management
CEO → COO → Oncology Administrator

Physician-Directed Management
CEO → COO → Oncology Medical Director → Oncology Administrator

Dyad Management
CEO → COO → Oncology Administrator / Oncology Medical Director

Administrative Director	Physician Leader	Dyad Leadership
Philosophy: A highly trained, experienced manager who understands the organizational, operational, and financial implications of running a successful service line is best equipped to lead these complex enterprises.	Philosophy: Physician leaders may be best prepared to ensure quality and safety, achieve patient outcome goals, pursue service development opportunities, and foster relationships with key physicians.	Philosophy: The benefits of having both the clinical expertise of a physician and the business experience of an administrator may outweigh the added complexity that accompanies a dyad leadership structure.
Benefits and Concerns	**Benefits and Concerns**	**Benefits and Concerns**
• An experienced administrator may have a better understanding of the business aspects related to service line organization and development. • It may be easier to facilitate effective communication between administrative staff and physicians. • The medical staff may relate better to a physician leader.	• Physicians have a unique understanding of the healthcare environment, which may result in improved patient outcomes and clinical coordination. • It may be easier to recruit top physician talent under this model. • It is difficult to find a physician leader who has business experience and can balance the clinical and management demands of the position.	• Each leader brings a specialized skill set to the organization, integrating a patient care and clinical focus with a hospital business focus. • A more effective line of communication is created between administrative and medical staff. • A dual reporting relationship introduces additional complexities into the system. • Lines of authority may blur, leading to confusion or inefficiencies.

Source: ECG Management Consultants, Inc.

The Importance of Governance and Leadership

The challenge is that the majority of cancer services are ambulatory and less connected to the traditional inpatient nursing functions. It can also be difficult to find suitable candidates with both an oncology nursing background and the management expertise needed to lead a complex service line.

Physician-directed model

Strong service lines often incorporate physician leadership in meaningful management positions to help solidify the service line and enhance hospital/physician alignment. The physician-directed model features a physician in the key leadership role charged with providing management and clinical oversight of the oncology service line. A key benefit is that a physician leader may be best prepared to ensure quality and safety, achieve pay-for-performance goals, pursue service development opportunities, and foster relationships with the employed physicians and independent medical staff members. Given that many leading cancer physicians hold administrative appointments, it also may be easier to recruit top physician talent under this model. However, in order to make this model successful, it is necessary to recruit a physician leader who has business experience and understands the nuances of running a highly complex organization. Balancing the demands of clinical oversight with the varying operational, political, and financial issues can create unrealistic demands on the individual and necessitate providing additional administrative support that reports to the physician leader.

Shared management (dyad) model

In recent years, many hospitals have begun to favor the shared management (dyad) structures, in which a physician is paired with an administrative leader. This construct directly engages physicians in the management of service line

Chapter 3

functions, which is one of the key goals of improving performance. The shared management or dyad model is powerful because it elevates the role of the physician, promoting alignment between providers and the hospital.

The dyad model combines aspects of the administrator-led and physician-directed models, pairing an administrator and physician to work in tandem to lead the service line. The service line benefits from this structure by having both the clinical expertise of a physician and the business experience of an administrator. Also, it may create a more effective line of communication between administrative, medical, and nursing staff.

However, there is a degree of added complexity that accompanies a dyad leadership structure because each leader's roles and responsibilities may not be clearly defined. The leaders' personalities may limit the effectiveness of the dyad model due to the lack of a clear line of authority. In most organizations, the dyad approach identifies the physician as the leader of the clinical service line, whereas the executive is accountable for finance and operations. This usually reduces confusion in the organization and between the leaders. Figure 3.4 illustrates the division of responsibilities between the dyad leaders.

The Importance of Governance and Leadership

FIGURE 3.4

DYAD LEADERSHIP RESPONSIBILITIES

Physician Leader
- Quality of care.
- Coordination of care across specialties/services.
- Product standardization/cost containment/resource utilization.
- Medical staff development.
- Research.
- Education.

(Overlap)
- Program development.
- Strategic and Business planning.
- Physician performance monitoring.
- Working with hospital leadership to outline organizationwide strategy.

Administrative Leader
- Resource allocation. Budgeting/oversight/financial control.
- Performance analysis/monitoring.
- Coordination with physician leadership.
- Coordination of administrative functions across facilities/locations.

Source: ECG Management Consultants, Inc.

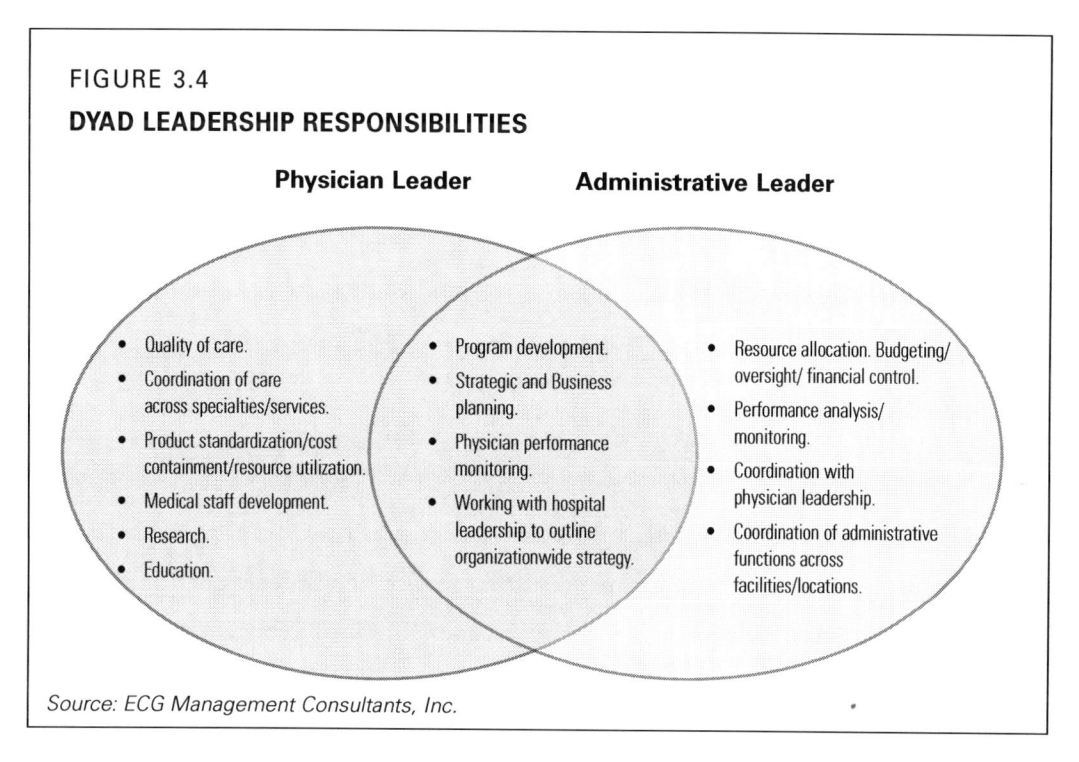

Although the management structures discussed previously are illustrated as sets of linked ovals in Figure 3.4, the reality is that the shapes represent human beings with strengths, weaknesses, and personalities that should be considered when selecting the right management construct. In one oncology service line, for example, a skilled clinician was selected to direct all cancer services. As the cancer program expanded, her lack of managerial expertise created operational and financial issues. With unfavorable budget performance and growing frustration among other physicians about the lack of growth and investment in new programs, the CEO recognized the need to create a dyad structure. The addition of a skilled administrator allowed the physician leader to focus on quality and provided the executive skills necessary to put the service line back on track. When evaluating

Chapter 3

alternative management approaches, it is important to assess the benefits and challenges of the options and implement structures that align with both the strategic goals of the service line and available leadership talents. Taking the time to develop and communicate clear expectations with regard to reporting relationships, roles, and responsibilities aids in creating accountability for each position. Additionally, the process of defining each position's function within the service line creates a framework for decision-making and implementation.

Managing Performance

Although integrated governance and management structures are the backbone of a successful service line, the performance of the service line is dependent on the ability of the organization to provide the right combination of people, data, and tools to enhance decision-making. When designing oncology service line governance and management structures, organizations typically focus their efforts on defining the numbers and types of positions and designing reporting relationships, often stopping short of developing the framework required for productive decision-making. To create an effective oncology service line, it is imperative that processes are in place for decision-making and implementation, and that performance can be measured and monitored for evaluation.

The old management adage "you can't manage what you don't measure" is especially applicable to oncology service line management. The complexity of cancer care, however, has made it particularly difficult to create meaningful quality and performance reports because cancer can be located in different organs, diagnosed and treated in different stages, and treated using different modalities. To determine

The Importance of Governance and Leadership

the financial impact of the oncology service line and its impact on quality and outcome measures, service line administrators need to set quantifiable goals and measure against them. The following guidelines should be considered when designing a performance monitoring process:

- Define financial, service, and quality goals for the service line by working collaboratively with key organizational and service line stakeholders

- Choose benchmarks that center around the patient, reflect industry standards, or are well recognized to avoid political backlash and encourage buy-in

- Build or invest in technologies that help quantify performance on a regular basis in order to develop a culture of accountability

- Continuously measure and communicate in an organized manner, so that everyone in the service line knows what is being measured and why

- Assign accountability for measuring and reporting accurate data in a timely manner to an individual or a group of individuals to ensure continuity in reporting

- Choose goals that are attainable and limit metrics to those that can be affected by changes in behavior to achieve service line-based performance improvement

With the recent trend toward pay-for-performance and quality-based incentives, industry sources such as the National Committee for Quality Assurance, the American College of Surgeon's CoC, the National Cancer Institute, and the Institute of Medicine have expanded the availability of best practice benchmarks

Chapter 3

to include outcomes, quality, and service. Figure 3.5 provides examples of commonly used performance metrics for oncology service lines.

FIGURE 3.5
EXAMPLE PERFORMANCE MEASURES

Metric	Measure
Service	
Patient satisfaction	Press Ganey Associates, Inc., general satisfaction report—percentage; other patient satisfaction reports (e.g., FAMCare, Hospital Consumer Assessment of Healthcare Providers and Systems)
Time from cancer detection to diagnosis	Days
Access to end-of-life care	Days from terminal diagnosis
Quality	
Survival rate by tumor site	Percentage
Clinician experience	Number of times a clinician performs a particular procedure in a year
Potentially preventable adverse events/healthcare-acquired conditions	Composite score (e.g., National Quality Forum [NQF] #531)[1]
Absence of chemotherapy errors	Percentage of treatments per month
Medication reconciliation	Percentage of postdischarge reconciliation within a month for patients age 65 years and older (e.g., NQF #554)
Pressure ulcers from care	Patient days
Radiation critical results reporting	Percentage reported same day
Accuracy with tumor staging protocols	Percentage of total
Screening for fall risk	Percentage of total
Process improvement initiative identification	Once
Process improvement initiative adherence	Quarterly
Operational/Financial	
Wait time for appointment scheduling	Days
Margin per case by site	Dollars per inpatient case; dollars per outpatient case or encounter
Market share	Percentage of total cancer services in primary service area; percentage of total cancer services in secondary service area
New patient growth	Number of consults and new patient encounters.
Annual fundraising endowment	Dollars per year

Composite score includes accidental puncture or laceration, iatrogenic pneumothorax, postoperative deep vein thrombosis or pulmonary embolism, postoperative wound dehiscence, decubitus ulcer, selected infections due to medical care, postoperative hip fracture, and postoperative sepsis.

Source: ECG Management Consultants, Inc.

Key Takeaways

Creating an integrated oncology service line governance and management structure is the first step to eliminating clinical silos and creating a disease-focused cancer delivery model that results in the best outcomes, quality, and experience for the patient. An integrated service line is also beneficial from a financial standpoint because it allows for better coordination and collaboration, which significantly increases an organization's ability to execute strategic and operational plans.

When developing an oncology service line structure, organizations should consider the following advice:

- Evaluate the level of integration that is needed across disease sites, disease stages, and treatment modalities to accomplish clinical, operational, and financial goals

- Develop governance and committee structures that include physicians and support the standardization of practice across the service line

- Understand the key influencers of change for stakeholders and incorporate them into the structure and decision-making process

- Invest time and effort into defining responsibilities, expectations, and reporting accountabilities for each position

Chapter 3

- Create the infrastructure needed to report timely performance metrics so that decisions can be based on fact

- Train staff on how to operate under new accountability, communicate effectively within the structure, and use performance metrics and monitoring to accomplish needed change

Reference

1. American College of Surgeons Commission on Cancer. (2011). *Cancer Program Standards 2012: Ensuring Patient-Centered Care.* Chicago: American College of Surgeons.

CHAPTER 4

Creating Aligned Physician Relationships

A quick search of almost every cancer center's marketing materials reveals a common phrase: "our coordinated approach to cancer care." The reality is that relatively few organizations have in fact attained the degree of alignment with physicians that is needed for true clinical coordination.

This chapter focuses on how to create aligned physician relationships, which are a critical aspect of building a coordinated cancer service line. There is little doubt regarding the clinical and programmatic benefits of aligning the various oncology specialties. However, several forces exist that have historically prevented or slowed alignment. Regulatory restrictions, such as the Stark Law and antitrust laws, often limit business relationships or create enough complexities that providers elect not to pursue greater alignment. Financial hurdles are particularly significant in cancer-related services, because many oncology providers rely on ancillary business for a large portion of their revenue. As providers seek greater alignment, the following questions often arise regarding how to preserve this income:

- How will ancillary services be consolidated across the various providers, and what will be the financial impact?

- How can the providers share in the financial success of the aligned organizations?

Chapter 4

In addition, the history of provider independence and the culture of private practice can create resistance to cooperative arrangements. There are several alignment models, all with unique benefits and limitations. Not surprisingly, the right model depends on the unique needs and goals of the organizations and physicians involved.

Affiliation Models

The physician alignment models shown in Figure 4.1 range from limited structures, such as part-time medical directorships that engage participants in a limited scope of oncology service line activities, to more comprehensive arrangements, including professional services agreements (PSA), comanagement arrangements, and employment, which can deeply involve oncology physicians in the leadership, development, and operations of all oncology services.

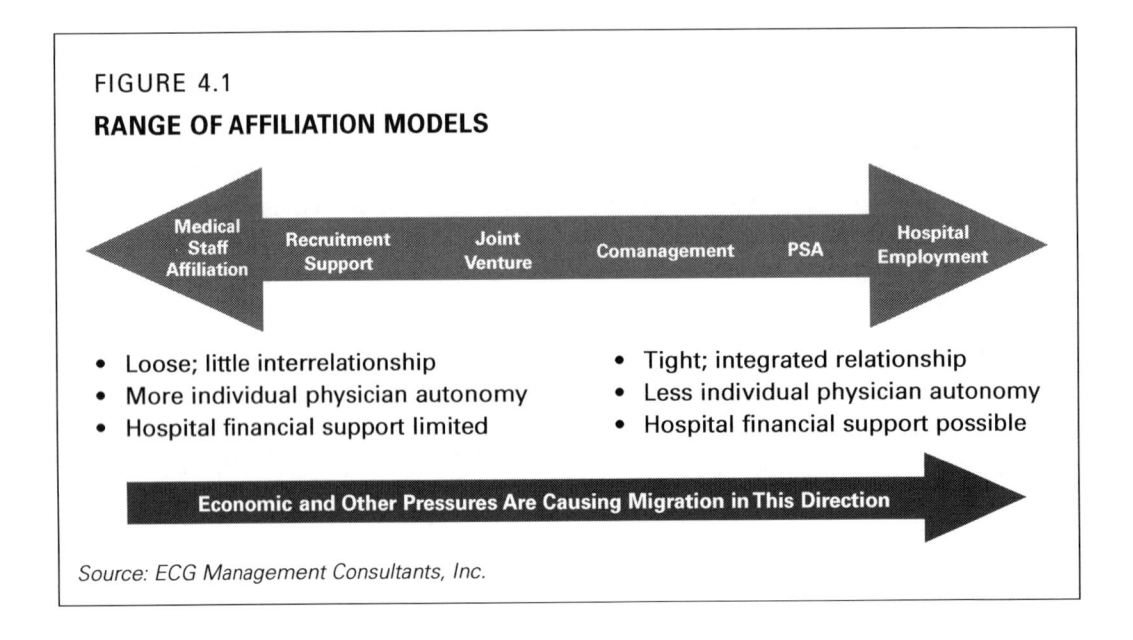

FIGURE 4.1
RANGE OF AFFILIATION MODELS

Medical Staff Affiliation — Recruitment Support — Joint Venture — Comanagement — PSA — Hospital Employment

- Loose; little interrelationship
- More individual physician autonomy
- Hospital financial support limited

- Tight; integrated relationship
- Less individual physician autonomy
- Hospital financial support possible

Economic and Other Pressures Are Causing Migration in This Direction

Source: ECG Management Consultants, Inc.

The correct alignment model for your situation is the one that addresses the unique needs of both the hospital and physicians and can be successfully implemented. Often, this involves initially adopting and layering multiple models that meet the specific requirements of individual physician groups or subspecialties, then revising them over time to address emerging needs. When weighing the options for physician alignment models, there are four key considerations: physician leadership, quality and service enhancement, strategic positioning, and flexibility.

Physician leadership

The success of the cancer service line will depend on physician leaders who have the ability to drive change. It is important to assess the leadership capabilities of participating physicians to identify physician champions who will direct the development and implementation of the service line strategy. In certain situations, organizations may recognize the need to bring in an outside physician leader; however, it is recommended that you first examine your existing physicians to determine if there are individuals who have the competency and desire to guide the process. If the existing physicians lack experience in leading broader organizational activities, the situation may warrant pursuing alignment strategies that are more focused on specific tumor-site programs (e.g., breast cancer) or for select specialties (e.g., medical oncology).

Quality and service enhancement

A principal goal of the service line should be to improve the delivery of patient care in terms of both clinical quality and patient service. To accomplish these objectives, the hospital should consider the coordination of services across the

Chapter 4

cancer care continuum, the support of clinical care teams, the organization of services that are centered on the patient, and the engagement of physicians with respect to driving clinical standardization. It is common that the more integrated relationships will be more effective than the loosely integrated models in programmatic redesign that will yield substantial results for enhancing patient access and operational efficiencies. Consideration of the impact of more integrated models on quality of care should typically be weighed against the financial and political ramifications. For example, if the organization has a culture driven by high-quality, low-cost care, it will likely need to pursue highly integrated alignment structures that engage physicians in the change management necessary to accomplish these goals. The direct financial terms of the relationship may stand out as more expensive to the hospital than alternative structures; however, the growth in market share and reductions in costs will likely result in net organizational gain.

Strategic positioning

To select the appropriate alignment model(s) for the cancer service line, it is important to assess the current and desired strategic positioning of your organization in the context of internal and external dimensions, such as development of a cancer center, formation of tumor-site–based institutes, expansion of research capabilities, and national accreditation. If the hospital already has established physician alignment pathways and protocols, these should guide the strategy for the oncology service line to ensure that there is a degree of consistency in how alignment is being pursued across the hospital. However, it is important that the health system reexamine the market dynamics in terms of the specific impact to oncology services and tailor the strategy appropriately. This includes understanding how certain models will impact other physicians' relationships with the hospital, what advantage may be gained with payer contracting, and how the structure will differentiate the hospital and aligned physicians compared to competitors.

For example, the physician alignment strategy may not produce an immediate increase in oncology market share, but it may forestall your competitor from gaining one. A market assessment could facilitate this process by identifying strategic opportunities for specific cancer services and tumor-site programs to help prioritize alignment opportunities. Each market factor will be critical to guiding discussions and limiting the exploration of alignment options to those that support the future direction of the hospital and physician group.

Flexibility
Physician alignment is a moving target. As changes continue in reimbursement and technology, the needs of physicians and hospitals will evolve. In some cases, the most prudent strategy may be to implement alignment models that are functional and possible today, with the goal of shifting to more tightly integrated models in the future. While flexibility is important to address physicians' concerns regarding compensation and control, a standardized approach to alignment models will generally enhance further integration.

Overview of potential models
Physician alignment models vary widely in cost, the degree of physician integration they foster, and strategic value to a hospital or healthcare system (see Figure 4.2). Each model presents both benefits and risks. Meeting strategic needs, improving physician integration, and mitigating financial risk for both physicians and the hospital are key considerations when evaluating alignment models.

Chapter 4

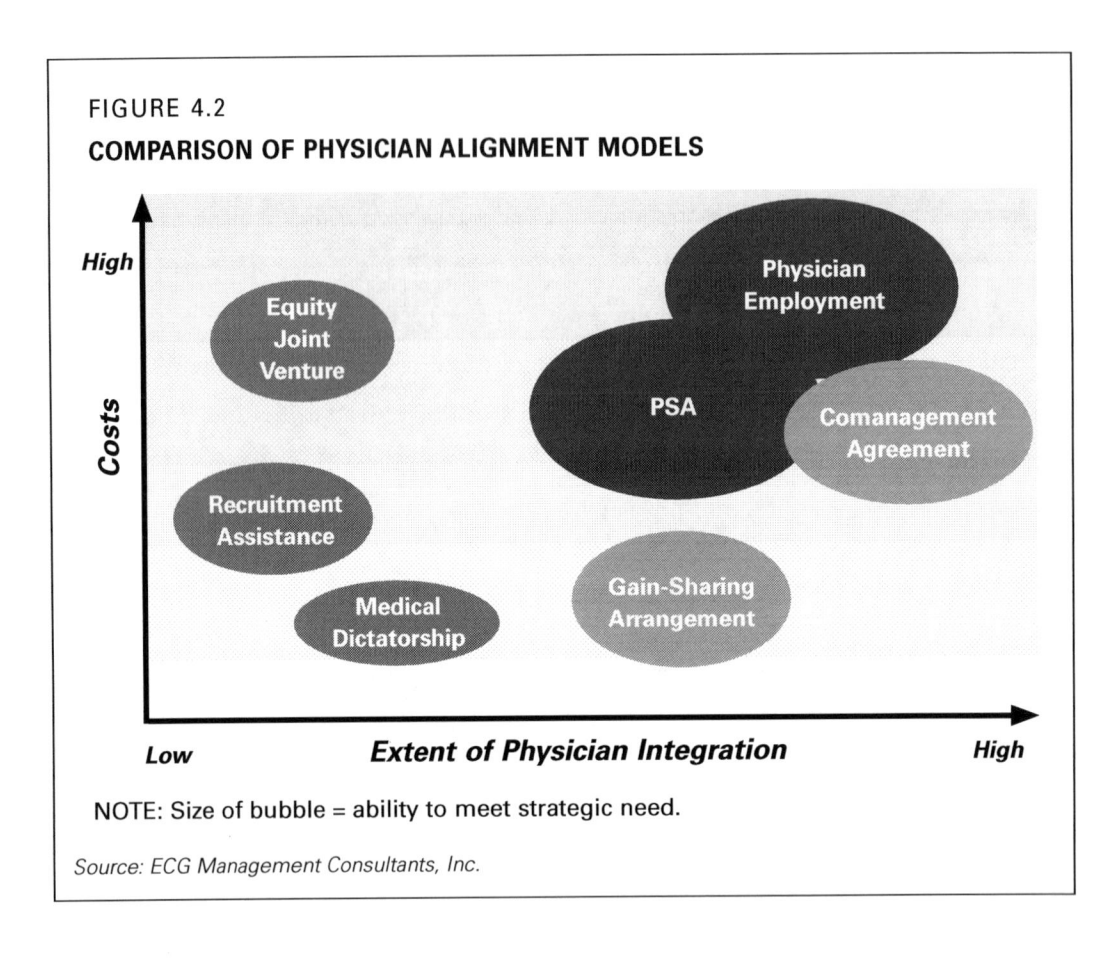

FIGURE 4.2
COMPARISON OF PHYSICIAN ALIGNMENT MODELS

[Bubble chart with axes: Costs (Low to High, vertical) and Extent of Physician Integration (Low to High, horizontal). Bubbles labeled: Equity Joint Venture, Physician Employment, PSA, Comanagement Agreement, Recruitment Assistance, Medical Dictatorship, Gain-Sharing Arrangement.]

NOTE: Size of bubble = ability to meet strategic need.

Source: ECG Management Consultants, Inc.

Hospitals have long offered independent physician groups recruiting assistance, primarily in the form of income guarantees for new physicians or aid in the recruitment process. The medical staff development plan should be used as a starting point for the determination of recruitment priorities and identification of practices for which recruitment assistance may be mutually beneficial.

Recruitment assistance

For those groups that are interested in recruiting, the hospital can then determine whether the provision of support is necessary. If the hospital is able to demonstrate that there is a deficit of physicians in a particular specialty through a community need assessment, then the hospital can recruit and place a new physician into the community and offer an income guarantee. Income guarantees are typically structured as forgivable loans with recourse to the group or the recruited physician in the event that the physician departs prior to fulfilling a multiyear service requirement. Alternatively, the hospital can aid physician groups in the recruiting process by providing help from hospital recruiters and giving candidates a welcoming experience.

The benefits of offering recruitment assistance are that it allows the hospital to continue to support independent physicians and does not require the financial commitment of other, more hardwired options. Having a private practice alternative enables new recruits to choose the environment in which they wish to practice. Recruitment assistance may also help reinforce positive relationships with the groups being assisted. Furthermore, an income guarantee gives the independent physician group time to help build the practice of the new physician, protecting physician compensation while the new recruit cultivates his or her patient base.

Many groups, however, do not find recruitment assistance enough to induce them to recruit. Income guarantees typically extend for only the first two to three years of practice. After this time, the new physician must be able to support his or her own practice; otherwise, the economics of all physicians in the group are affected. Particularly in smaller groups, physicians face the concern that their income will

Chapter 4

be cut and their patient base cannibalized by adding a new physician. While it may be in the strategic interest of the hospital to recruit to increase access to care and grow services, motivating private physician practices to do so can be difficult. As this demonstrates, fundamentally, recruitment assistance on its own does not necessarily align physician incentives with hospital incentives, so it generally needs to be used in conjunction with other alignment tools.

Another issue with recruitment assistance is the current regulatory constraint that prohibits the group from imposing restrictive covenants on the new physician. Groups are understandably reluctant to take on a new physician and help him or her establish a healthy practice if that physician has no restriction on competing with the group if the arrangement does not work out. A further dilemma in recruiting arrangements is that the hospital cannot provide support to the group to cover overhead expenses unless they are new costs necessitated by a new physician. Consulting legal counsel regarding these restrictions, as well as the regulatory and legal issues regarding any alignment model, is warranted.

Placement of a hospital-employed physician in an independent group

An alternative to a recruiting arrangement is the placement of a new physician who has been hired by the hospital into an established medical practice. This option avoids some of the regulatory constraints of recruitment assistance and allows the hospital to pay for the employed physician's use of space and overhead. Also, in this type of arrangement, there is no recourse to the physician or the group if the physician leaves prior to fulfilling a service requirement, because these arrangements are structured as employment agreements. Ensuring group cohesion can prove challenging; however, these arrangements do allow the physician to build a practice within the parameters of a group and, in many instances, result in the physician joining the group at the end of the employment period.

Medical directorship

Medical directorships are a common means to involve physicians in hospital administrative roles. However, to be an effective physician alignment tool, they should be carefully structured so physicians will have the proper incentives to attain hospital and service line goals. As physicians come under increasing reimbursement pressure, they are more likely to require compensation for participating in activities that were once considered voluntary duties, including medical staff administration, quality improvement, and peer review.

Paying independent physicians as part-time medical directors to provide these services is one way to encourage participation and engage them in service line planning and management. Most hospitals have historically utilized medical directorships, such as chiefs of oncology or service line directors, as a means to engage physicians and perhaps to give them an alternate revenue stream. However, these relationships are being reexamined, both to ensure that the agreements meet legal requirements and to drive active participation in the service line. Increasingly, medical directorships are being redesigned to include specific roles and responsibilities that enhance service line function and include incentive-based payments.

Under an enhanced medical directorship arrangement, physicians may become part-time employees of the hospital or remain as independent contractors for the portion of their time spent conducting medical directorship duties, which include the following:

Chapter 4

- Specific roles and responsibilities for the fixed portion of the contract typically relate to:

  - Clinical oversight

  - Quality improvement initiatives

  - Involvement in hospital and service line committees

  - Provision of leadership for strategic service line activities

  - Clinical research oversight

- Specific metrics used to reward the variable portion of the agreement could include:

  - Improvements in patient satisfaction scores

  - Achievement of specific quality/outcomes management goals, such as improvements in patient outcomes and compliance with Centers for Medicare & Medicaid Services or American College of Surgeons (ACoS) core measures

  - Achievement of strategic programmatic goals, such as recruitment of new physicians, presentations to the community, and timely development of a new strategic plan within a specified time period

  - Improvements in operational efficiency, such as enhanced clinical protocols

An advantage of paid medical directorships is that they can improve quality and care coordination through greater physician involvement in program design and oversight. The roles and responsibilities of medical directors usually leverage physicians' skill sets related to clinical expertise and programmatic development. Involving medical directors who are respected clinicians can improve compliance with new initiatives and drive support of service line strategies. Tailoring roles and responsibilities of medical directors to meet service line needs and using a compensation methodology that encompasses both fixed and variable components can help ensure that the hospital is realizing benefits from these positions. These directorships can also be implemented in a relatively short time frame with low startup costs.

For physicians to succeed as medical directors, they need to be able to separate their position as a leader of their physician group from their role as a representative of the hospital. In other words, they need to be able to wear two hats, which can be difficult for some physicians. Choosing medical directors can be a highly politicized and polarizing process. Physicians from rival groups may see the appointment of a physician from the opposing group as a show of favoritism by the hospital. Selected medical directors should be individuals who are well-respected members of the medical staff and who can bridge divides that often occur between physicians, particularly among independent physician groups. Changing and retooling existing directorships can also be difficult. Overall, medical directorships can be designed to be supportive of service line goals, but they represent an alignment tool that is best utilized in conjunction with other models of relationship building.

Chapter 4

Gain-sharing arrangement

Office of Inspector General (OIG)–approved gain-sharing arrangements entail the hospital sharing cost savings with associated physicians under an approved structure. Under these arrangements, the hospital pays the associated physicians a portion of the cost savings (historical costs less actual costs) directly attributable to specific changes in quality improvement. Payments are made to the physicians on a per capita basis. The hospital hires a program administrator to study historical practices and identify specific cost-saving opportunities. The hospital and physicians review and adopt recommendations as medically appropriate. Cost savings are calculated separately for each recommendation to preclude expense shifting. A "floor" is established for expected savings with no credit below the floor. There is no sharing of cost savings resulting from additional procedures, and contract term extensions are expected to incorporate updated base-year costs. To satisfy requirements, there must be no steering of costly patients to other hospitals, and this must be monitored through study of case severity, patient ages, and payers. Also, the arrangement must be disclosed to patients in writing.

The advantage of a gain-sharing arrangement is that it explicitly aligns physician and hospital financial incentives in pursuit of predetermined cost and quality goals. This promotes integration by directly involving physicians in establishing the goals and making program improvements such as protocol adjustments to meet them, and holding these physicians accountable for the results. It also is a step in preparing the hospital for value-based reimbursement trends.

However, gain-sharing arrangements have many disadvantages. One is that they are subject to close scrutiny by the OIG, which has approved only a few gain-sharing structures. Creating a gain-sharing arrangement that meets governmental requirements requires expert legal guidance, as well as administrative infrastructure to ensure that the metrics are tracked and documented appropriately. Gain-sharing arrangements can also have limited appeal to physicians, because the metrics used are somewhat narrow in focus and may not provide the degree of economic support desired.

Equity joint venture

Equity joint ventures are arrangements in which physicians and the hospital create a separate entity whereby they both invest and hold ownership stakes to provide clinical equipment or services. As the name suggests, equity joint ventures involve selling physicians a share of an entity that earns technical revenue. The physicians' ownership position is often combined with significant physician control of day-to-day operations, staffing, and scheduling.

Several types of joint ventures currently exist:

- Clinical equity joint venture: Under a clinical joint venture, the new business entity would provide, bill, and collect for all clinical and technical services

- Equipment equity joint venture: The new business entity (potentially co-owned by the hospital) typically leases equipment to the hospital, which would then provide, bill, and collect for clinical services

- Real estate equity joint venture: Similar to an equipment equity joint venture, the new business entity would own (and potentially manage) medical office space

Chapter 4

While these arrangements have historically been fairly common, clinical joint ventures have become less easy to administer in recent years due to increasingly restrictive regulations. Stark regulations state that any physician who has a financial relationship (e.g., ownership, investment, or receives compensation) with an entity cannot refer designated health services (DHS) to the entity and the entity cannot bill for the DHS referrals unless there is a qualifying exemption in place. Notably, radiation oncology services, as well as chemotherapy and many imaging modalities, are considered DHS. Stark regulations, along with the anti-kickback law, discourage volume-based payment mechanisms for DHS and have banned certain types of joint venture arrangements (e.g., per click leasing agreement) that reward physician stakeholders for increased volumes. Therefore, recent trends in oncology have seen an increase in equipment and real estate joint ventures and a decrease in clinical joint ventures.

If an organization is to develop a joint venture, the following should be kept in mind:

- If an existing business is converted to a joint venture, it must be purchased by the venture at fair market value (FMV).

- The joint venture should be governed by a board with representatives from both parties.

- In the case of equity joint ventures, as illustrated in Figure 4.3, economic distributions should be based on a member's percentage ownership interests in the joint venture (i.e., capital investments, rather than volume or referrals).

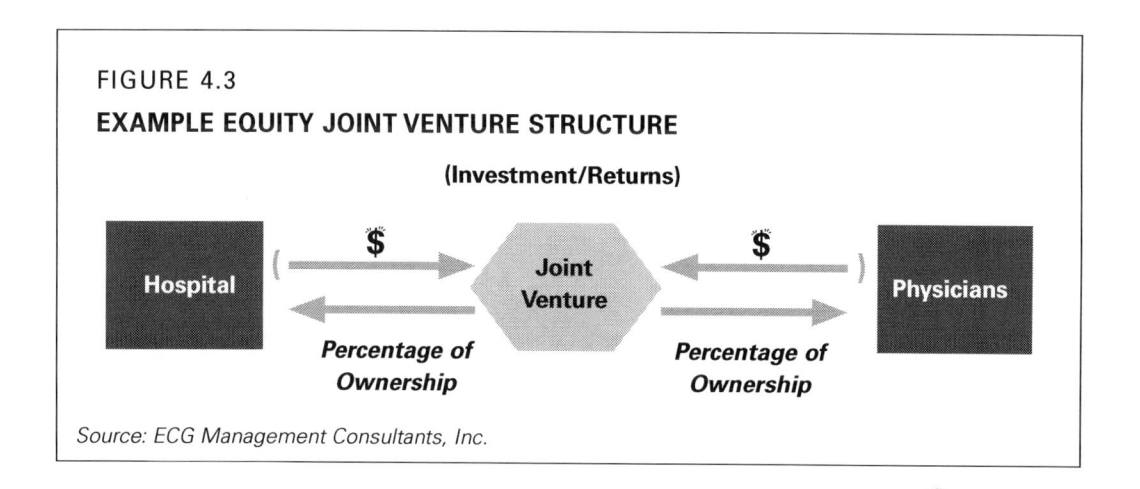

FIGURE 4.3
EXAMPLE EQUITY JOINT VENTURE STRUCTURE
(Investment/Returns)

Hospital → $ → Joint Venture ← $ ← Physicians

Percentage of Ownership | Percentage of Ownership

Source: ECG Management Consultants, Inc.

The chief benefit of a joint venture to the hospital is that through aligned incentives, it supports collaboration and economic alignment between the hospital and physicians. It gives the two parties an opportunity to work together as business partners and enhance their relationship. Given that the returns from these arrangements can be sizable, it also provides a means to enhance the economics of the physicians' practice.

For physicians, an equity joint venture diversifies revenue. It can also secure a strong market advantage by making the hospital a partner instead of an adversary. Given that both parties have seats on the entity's board, it also enables physician input for the facility's operation.

With any joint venture, several challenges must be addressed and factored into the decision prior to implementation. First, for the hospital, the joint venture can represent a loss of income, and increased volume from the new entity may not be sufficient to recover lost technical revenue.

Chapter 4

Reimbursement for outpatient services in a freestanding setting may also be lower, resulting in less revenue than if identical procedures were performed in the hospital. That being said, effective communication with physicians, careful construction of the joint venture, and early inclusion of legal counsel can help to mitigate many of the common risks.

CASE STUDY: Economic alignment through an equipment joint venture

The challenge
Numerous providers are involved in supplying comprehensive cancer care, and more often than not, they are in separate businesses. It is not uncommon to have a radiation oncology group, a medical oncology group, a radiology group, and a larger multispecialty group that all contribute to delivering cancer care. The fragmentation of business interests, not to mention different practice locations, creates barriers to developing a coordinated approach to care.

The situation
A 400-bed hospital wanted to develop a more comprehensive cancer center. The hospital believed that services were fragmented across various providers and difficult for most patients to navigate. Further, the hospital was committed to building a new cancer center. Three of the largest cancer-related groups in the community (a radiation oncology group, a medical oncology group, and a multispecialty group with medical oncologists and surgical oncologists) wanted to improve alignment and care coordination, but had competing business interests.

> **CASE STUDY**

Economic alignment through an equipment joint venture (cont.)

The solution
The three groups developed an equipment leasing joint venture. The joint venture owned much of the major equipment used in diagnosis and the delivery of cancer services (linear accelerators, PET/CT, etc.) and leased the equipment to the hospital. Profits resulting from the leasing arrangement were distributed to the joint venture members based on their ownership percentage. In addition, each member relocated its services to the new cancer center, thus enabling all cancer services to be offered in the same location—albeit by different providers.

The benefits
While the financial benefits have been reasonable—for example, consistent with the current market rate for medical equipment leasing companies—the real benefit has been the collaborative planning spurred by the economic alignment. The joint venture established an equipment review committee, thus ensuring that all providers were supportive of new technologies and their associated clinical programs. This degree of planning and interaction did not occur prior to the joint venture. In addition, the hospital's development of a new cancer facility paved the way for the various providers to colocate all cancer services within the same building. In the end, the physician groups were able to maintain their independence yet achieve enough economic alignment to support broader integration and collaboration initiatives.

Chapter 4

Comanagement agreement

Under a comanagement agreement, physicians and the hospital form a joint venture management company for the purpose of providing management services for the oncology service line or specific elements of the service line, such as the infusion center. The management company works in conjunction with oncology program administration to lead the service line and implement strategies. The management company enters into subcontracts with individual physician members to serve as medical directors and potentially employ the program administrator. The scope of the services required from program management determines the breadth of the management agreement and the fees associated with management services. The management company, through its designated physician leaders, provides administrative, medical directorship, and quality improvement services, as negotiated by the management company. The ownership of the management company and distributions are based on the capital contributed to the venture. Capitalized expenses, including a portion of startup fees and the value of any equipment, are included in the company.

Functions of the new management company may include:

- Actively managing the infusion center

- Advising on and implementing measures to improve the quality of service

- Advising on and implementing operational efficiencies and performance improvement in the delivery of service

- Developing and implementing plans to enhance efficiency of resource use that would standardize supply chain elements and staffing

- Working with the hospital to establish and facilitate the creation of standard service line scorecards and evidence-based practice guidelines

A fee is paid to the management company, composed of a fixed portion and a performance-based portion. The fixed portion would be based on the FMV of standard services rendered. The performance-based portion would be a set amount, determined in advance at the beginning of each contract year, which would be paid based on meeting specific quality and efficiency goals (such as performance with respect to core measures, maintenance of ACoS quality indicators, adherence to prescription procedures, and increased patient satisfaction). It is worth noting that within the management company, there are no passive investors—all physician partners are expected to be in a strong leadership role or at least be actively involved in the delivery of patient care.

The comanagement entity typically employs or leases the service line administrator, medical directors, and other management and administrative personnel. The service line pays a fee to the comanagement entity based on the FMV of management services, plus a bonus based on achievement of predetermined performance goals. The entity is governed by a board representing physicians and the hospital, and the profits are split in proportion to the ownership stakes of the shareholders (see Figure 4.4).

Chapter 4

FIGURE 4.4

EXAMPLE COMANAGEMENT MODEL STRUCTURE

```
                    ┌─────────────────────────────────┐
                    │    Hospital Governing Board     │
                    └─────────────────────────────────┘
                                    │
  ┌──────────────────┐    Management            ┌──────────────┐
  │Oncology Physician│    Company Reports       │   Hospital   │
  │    Investors     │    to Hospital Board     │              │
  └──────────────────┘                          └──────────────┘
          │      Appropriate      Appropriate Physician/Hospital
          │      Equity Split         Governance Split
  Payment Passed Through    ┌──────────────────────────┐
  to Physician Investors    │ Management Company, LLC  │◄── Management Fee:
                            └──────────────────────────┘    50% Fixed, 50% Based on
                                        │                   Performance Incentives
                            ┌──────────────────────────┐
                            │   Oncology Service Line  │
                            └──────────────────────────┘
```

Source: ECG Management Consultants, Inc.

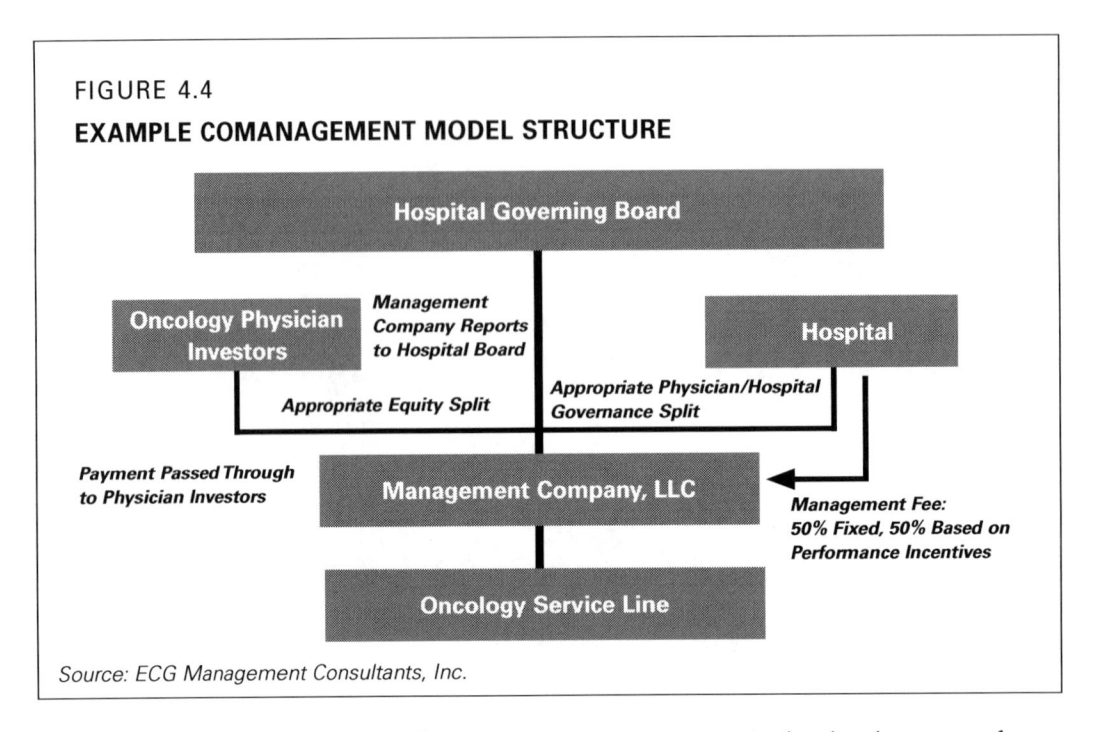

A variation of the traditional comanagement agreement is the development of a more limited agreement to have physicians aid in implementing select service line initiatives. Instead of establishing a joint venture for the management of the oncology service line, in this alternative, the new company is tasked with implementing specific initiatives to leverage the physicians' skill set, and physicians receive an FMV payment for their services. For instance, the physicians could be charged with developing standard-of-care protocols or exploring outreach opportunities. These initiatives should be strategic in nature and aid in achieving the service line's overall goals. The benefit of this is that it provides an opportunity to work together and determine if it is an endeavor that the two parties would like to continue on an expanded basis. Consulting arrangements for relevant services are generally straightforward and are typically limited in scope and of short duration.

The major benefit of comanagement is that physicians become partners with the hospital in driving programmatic development. Also, in this structure, physician managers are in a favorable position to enhance coordination of care. A great deal of control is ceded to the management company, giving it the ability to make significant positive changes. Financially, physicians can benefit from upside potential if they are able to achieve performance goals with the management company.

One of the key challenges is that a comanagement agreement requires physicians to be willing to dedicate significant time to managing the service line, which affects availability of time for patient care services. Since it is often difficult to compensate physicians for these services at a rate that is commensurate with their clinical and/or ancillary reimbursement, it can be difficult to attract enough physicians to successfully implement this type of arrangement. Going forward with a comanagement agreement may be more appropriate after the oncology service line strategy has been developed and physician leaders have been identified. Regardless, it can take six months or more to establish and implement a comanagement agreement, and these types of arrangements should be carefully reviewed by legal counsel.

PSA

A PSA is similar in structure to the foundation model frequently used in states, such as California and Texas, that restrict the employment of physicians by hospitals. Typically, a group or groups of physicians are linked to a hospital through a PSA, which is a contract that requires specific clinical and perhaps administrative services for an agreed-upon level of remuneration. PSAs are frequently tied to agreements whereby the physician group also supplies management services. PSAs can be simple or elaborate depending on the scope of services provided under the arrangement.

Chapter 4

Some organizations use a PSA model to mimic the economics of an employment type of arrangement when employment is not optimal. Often these arrangements are sought due to corporate practices in the local jurisdiction or physicians' desire to maintain some of their independence as well as a way out of the arrangement. Due to changes in reimbursement and/or financial performance, there is also an increasing trend among multispecialty groups to structure a PSA between a hospital and a particular specialty. Figure 4.5 illustrates a typical PSA structure.

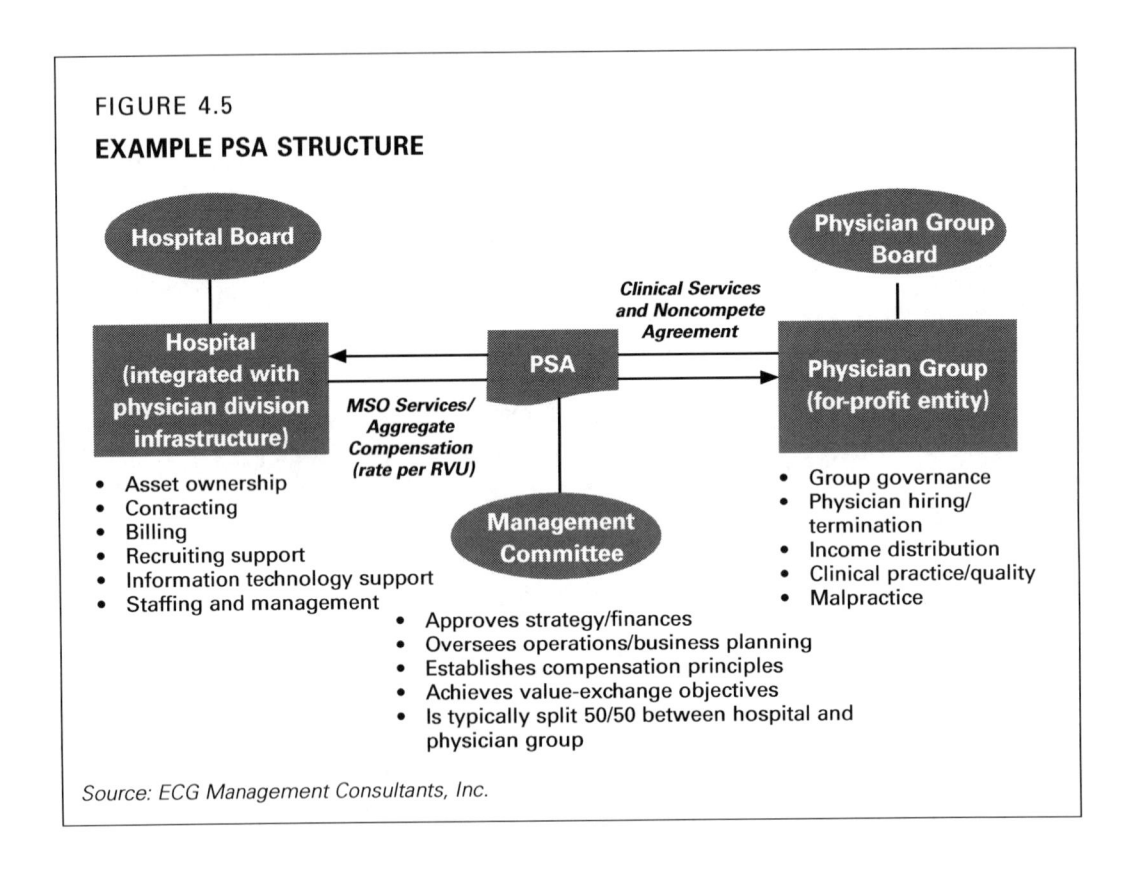

FIGURE 4.5
EXAMPLE PSA STRUCTURE

Hospital Board — **Hospital (integrated with physician division infrastructure)**
- Asset ownership
- Contracting
- Billing
- Recruiting support
- Information technology support
- Staffing and management

PSA
- Clinical Services and Noncompete Agreement
- MSO Services/Aggregate Compensation (rate per RVU)

Physician Group Board — **Physician Group (for-profit entity)**
- Group governance
- Physician hiring/termination
- Income distribution
- Clinical practice/quality
- Malpractice

Management Committee
- Approves strategy/finances
- Oversees operations/business planning
- Establishes compensation principles
- Achieves value-exchange objectives
- Is typically split 50/50 between hospital and physician group

Source: ECG Management Consultants, Inc.

PSAs are appealing because they create strong, coordinated relationships while allowing physicians to remain independent. In some instances, they are the first step before employment. They are also flexible, in that the services covered and the terms involved can be tailored to fit the circumstances. On the downside, PSAs are often very complex documents that require time for proper setup and legal review. PSAs also necessitate a degree of hospital infrastructure to be able to support and administer the contract. Because PSAs often involve some level of management service support by the physician group, they can result in duplicative services (e.g., information technology and billing) that impact operational efficiency. This type of vehicle is often chosen by organizations that want and are willing to invest in a tightly integrated physician group but encounter physician resistance to employment. To ensure successful integration, though, it is important to tailor an arrangement that not only creates aligned incentives but also promotes physician leadership through joint service line management and/or governance.

CASE STUDY

Economic alignment through a PSA

The challenge

Economic pressures continue to mount for physician groups, yet most oncologists still rely on chemotherapy drugs as a major financial contributor to their practice. Meanwhile, patients are seeking a more coordinated approach to care with less fragmentation among oncology providers and hospitals.

Chapter 4

> **CASE STUDY**
>
> ## Economic alignment through a PSA (cont.)
>
> ### The situation
> A 300-bed hospital and a local physician group teamed up to address the problem. The hospital qualified for 340B Drug Pricing Program rates and thus had the ability to acquire pharmaceuticals at a substantial discount. However, the group was reticent to give up chemotherapy business, as it historically represented a significant percentage of its compensation.
>
> ### The solution
> The hospital and the group entered into a PSA that leveraged the strengths of both organizations. The hospital became the provider of chemotherapy services, billing and collecting fees to and from Medicare and other payers. The hospital leased the physician group's chemotherapy space, which it converted to an outpatient department of the hospital. The physicians performed professional medical oncology services, as well as medical directorship duties for chemotherapy services. Under the terms of the agreement, the hospital contracted for full-time coverage of the infusion clinic at a flat rate. The payment included fees for both the physicians' professional time and the infrastructure leased from the group. The key benefit of the model was that it effectively transferred the physicians' downside economic risk to the hospital. However, in so doing, the physicians also gave up the upside economic opportunity due to the fixed payment structure.
>
> ### The benefits
> The benefits of the arrangement have been numerous. The economics and associated risk model make business sense for both the hospital and the physician group. In addition, there is greater economic alignment, and the framework now exists to build further integration among the various subspecialties.

Creating Aligned Physician Relationships

Physician employment

Employment potentially gives the service line and system the most control and the greatest integration with physicians. However, employment is also flexible; it can be structured in multiple ways to achieve many ends. These frameworks include maintaining multiple small groups and creating subspecialty pods, institutes, or fully integrated multispecialty groups. Reimbursement arrangements with individual physicians in the groups can also range from productivity-based payment to methods that include incentives for participation in management, quality improvement, and care coordination activity.

Employment is often the preferred model for physicians facing reimbursement cuts and higher operating costs. It also appeals to younger physicians, who generally seek a more equal work-life balance than their older colleagues. Increasingly, employment is becoming a practical necessity to keep physicians in place and to recruit new physicians.

Employing oncologists also presents a variety of challenges, including maintaining financial viability and potentially alienating independent physicians. To fully integrate physicians with service line operations, employment requires significant investment in practice management and support infrastructure; therefore, the employed practice may never break even on operations. This is particularly true within organizations that either do not benefit from reimbursement gains (due to provider-based and/or hospital rates) or do not qualify for reduced 340B pricing. Because the financial and strategic risk is high, employment arrangements must be carefully structured to promote productivity and ongoing physician participation in service line governance.

Chapter 4

Physician Alignment Planning Process

The planning process for creating aligned physician relationships in oncology is similar to the process outlined in Chapter 2. The process should be deliberate and facilitated in such a way that it results in a structure that is both effective and attainable, given your unique situation. There should be a clear progression from vision to goals to strategies to tactics. A steering committee should be created with senior leadership representation from both the hospital and the physician practices, and standing meetings should be scheduled on a routine basis. The following is a summary of seven key steps in a physician alignment planning process.

Agree on a work plan

The first step is to agree on a work plan that is both transparent and comprehensive. The work plan details how the hospital and physicians will reach agreement and will describe the various elements of analysis that need to be completed. The work plan will specify the timelines for interviews, data collection, practice reviews, and consideration of alternatives, among others. This will serve as the road map to guide affiliation planning and will ensure that there are no surprises along the way for either the hospital or physicians.

Gather input from stakeholders

A critical part of the planning process is for both hospital leadership and physician stakeholders to independently determine their vision of an optimal alignment structure and what they hope to accomplish. This is best done by interviewing key leaders and reporting back to the steering committee regarding similarities and differences of the participants. Far too often, organizations are well along in a planning process only to realize that they are not on the same page with respect to the options under consideration. Given findings of the interview process, the next step is to have a focused dialogue that will help each party gain an understanding of the other's motivating factors and goals that must be respected in any affiliation arrangement. It should be remembered that in addition to financial arrangements, strategic, operational, and cultural concerns must be addressed. Each physician who is considering affiliation with the hospital should be engaged in this dialogue in order to gain a clear understanding the unique issues and perspectives of all potential participants.

Establish a shared direction

The vision and goals of potential alignment must be addressed from the onset of planning. Both the hospital and physicians should discuss independently what they hope to achieve through alignment. In most cases, it is relatively easy for the hospital to articulate what alignment with physicians would entail and what it hopes to accomplish. For the physicians, on the other hand, there is often considerable diversity in both how affiliation would be structured and what benefits would be realized. It is useful to have these differences among physicians clearly identified because doing so can help determine which goals are most important and move the group toward consensus. In addition, for the hospital, the process can help with carefully considering the implications of different alignment structures and ensuring that the senior leadership team agrees on a preferred approach. The following key questions should be addressed:

- What are the desired attributes of an alignment model?

- What are barriers from each party's perspective?

Chapter 4

- How will alignment facilitate the organization's overall vision for oncology care in its market?

- Which structures for oncology best support the hospital's broader physician alignment strategy?

- How will alignment support the community need for oncology services and subspecialty care?

Conduct initial feasibility analysis and evaluate options
The hospital, working with physician leadership, should then consider the goals and objectives of both parties and determine the alternative structures they recommend for further consideration. Each alternative should be evaluated using an explicit set of criteria, including:

- Fit with overall hospital/system strategy

- Ability to accomplish patient care goals

- Ability to meet physician objectives

- Financial implications, including one-time and ongoing expenses

- Administrative burden

This process will help facilitate a dialogue among leadership and will provide necessary information and perspective to interested physicians. During this step, major terms, as well as any items for resolution through ongoing research, analysis, discussions, and/or negotiations, should be documented.

Present models and facilitate decision-making process

The dialogue with the physicians should continue with the review of specific models for alignment between physicians and the hospital. Each model under consideration should be presented in terms of goals and limitations, the mechanics of how it works, the potential financial implications, and the benefits and requirements. Discussing the specific issues related to governance, management, structure, operations, economics, and so forth will be critical to ensuring a complete understanding of the alternatives. Drafting a detailed conceptual model of the preferred arrangement(s) is often helpful in revealing and resolving key issues. This is generally a narrative-type document with considerable specificity, rather than a high-level Microsoft® PowerPoint® document, because such presentations often lead to ambiguity. Facilitating a conversation with the physicians regarding which models they would like to further investigate is the crucial component of this step.

Address financial implications

Early in the planning process, the hospital should analyze the financial implications to better understand which models maximize the collective resources of the parties and generate the most favorable return on investment. Building the pro forma and understanding the business case and financial ramifications are critical in deciding which alignment models are feasible and in forecasting any budgetary impacts. Each model requires a varying degree of capital investment, and the specific terms of the arrangements will have a significant impact on the operating margins going forward. Therefore, it is recommended that the financial modeling begin early in the development process to ensure that deals are structured in a way that maintains sustainability. In addition, the financial modeling process will allow the parties to understand the financial trade-offs related to physician

Chapter 4

compensation, physician recruitment and practice growth, reimbursement changes, capital budgeting, and practice acquisition values. The financial model should also evaluate the overall organizational impact of any new economic relationships. For example, if a hospital elects to structure a comanagement arrangement with a group of medical oncologists, the hospital should analyze the potential impact that the relationship will have on reducing the hospital's operating costs and changing utilization patterns.

Craft key terms

Depending on the model being pursued, the specific terms of an agreement will differ. In all cases, however, consensus must be obtained and legal review completed. A variety of analyses and activities are required to reach a mutually agreeable term sheet and/or subsequent letter of intent. Many of the decisions, analyses, and terms relate specifically to economic alignment and will not be applicable to every model (e.g., practice valuation). Figure 4.6 summarizes the range of decision-making and supporting activity that may need to be completed prior to implementing an alignment model.

FIGURE 4.6
WHAT TO COMPLETE BEFORE IMPLEMENTING AN ALIGNMENT MODEL

Decision	Supporting Activity/Analysis
Guiding principles	• Development of draft principles, goals, and objectives • Confirmation of overall working vision
Governance, management, organizational, and legal structures	• Development of structural options and key terms
Ancillary services solution	• Assessment regarding provision of services • Preliminary valuation of ancillary business (if applicable)
Physician compensation, benefits, and employment considerations (if applicable)	• Current physician compensation and benefits • Proposed physician compensation and benefits (e.g., rates, payment methodologies, incentives)
Summary of transaction structure and payment terms	• Transaction type and included/excluded assets and liabilities • Impact of various physician initiatives • Preliminary valuation of practice assets, including any ancillary services (if applicable) • Viability of practice as a stand-alone entity (if applicable) • Acquirer debt capacity and capital structure (if applicable) • Tax implications from acquisition (if applicable)

Source: ECG Management Consultants, Inc.

Key Takeaways

Hospitals and physicians are increasingly focusing on alignment as a strategy to deliver more integrated patient care and ensure a competitive advantage in today's healthcare market. Appropriately structured, all of these alignment arrangements can facilitate the development of a more coordinated cancer program or service line. The types of models used by organizations range widely and ultimately depend on the unique needs of each party. Regardless, it is important to evaluate

Chapter 4

and design a model with the support of legal counsel to ensure that it complies with the ever-changing rules and regulations associated with these types of relationships. In summary, the following advice should be considered when developing aligned physician relationships:

- An overall strategy for physician alignment needs to be created that promotes the hospital's mission and values

- Physicians and administration should be involved in the planning process to ensure that the needs of both parties are met

- While a standardized approach to alignment may be the hospital's overarching goal, strategies should be designed with flexibility due to the continuously changing balance of power among physician groups, hospitals, and other providers

- Organizations often adopt multiple alignment models and/or initiatives to meet the specific needs of the service line's physician groups and specialties

- In choosing a model, the parties should consider its impact on all clinical and operating processes related to the coordination of oncology services

- The strategic benefits should be weighed against the financial and political ramifications of alignment to ensure a long-term, financially viable partnership

- Regardless of the alignment model(s) chosen, it is important to ensure that appropriate infrastructure can be built to ultimately operationalize the arrangement

CHAPTER 5

Key Elements of a Successful Oncology Transaction

Having completed the initial physician alignment planning, hospital and physician leadership are ready to begin defining the details of the arrangement. While the parties may agree on an overall approach, the negotiation of transaction details can reveal challenges and disagreements that will need resolution. Taking the time to systematically work through the various deal points is critical to long-term success; however, it is not unusual for hospitals to rush the transaction process to meet a perceived crisis or artificial deadline. It is in these situations that obstacles can emerge that may disrupt negotiations and ultimately stall or derail the transaction process.

Ultimately, the details of the alignment model must reflect the unique needs of the players and the particular market. Despite their range in design and complexity, transactions that are successfully completed typically utilize a fairly standard method to work through the various issues and deal points. This chapter outlines an effective process for these discussions and highlight the key trends that have emerged in oncology transactions.

Chapter 5

Definition of the Transaction Goals

Cancer programs and physicians should focus on defining critical success factors for the transaction. Most importantly, the oncology program and the physicians will need to establish how physicians will be rewarded for their contributions. For example, hospitals frequently see acquisitions as part of a strategy to expand services available to the community and enhance or protect market share. Compare this to medical groups' dominant objective of protecting the compensation and lifestyle of their physician shareholders. Reaching concurrence on both shared and unilateral objectives will ensure that both parties' needs can be met.

The transaction goals and objectives, in combination with the affiliation objectives (defined in Chapter 4), will serve as the evaluation criteria to determine an appropriate model and can also help guide the first discussions. However, it is important to expand on these initial objectives when evaluating what each party hopes to achieve through the actual transaction negotiation. For example, physicians may have disparate opinions about the level of risk or types of incentives they want in their compensation plan, while the hospital has limitations on the types of compensation models that can be used legally. Regardless, it is important to determine which terms are most important to each party before engaging in detailed discussions. Depending on the group's particular dynamics, this process could be initiated through individual stakeholder interviews or focus groups and then shared with a broader steering committee of hospital and physician representatives; alternatively, the committee could jointly evaluate its goals for alignment. Thinking through the various issues early on will help frame the discussion and ensure that there is consensus on an overall shared direction. If consensus cannot be reached on vision and priorities for the relationship, it makes sense to explore alternatives to affiliation discussions.

Evaluate Business Implications

Once the objectives of the transaction are agreed to, organizations tend to rush through negotiations in an attempt to quickly finalize an agreement. Even in the most urgent circumstances, it is important to utilize a structured process that will facilitate informed and shared decision-making while avoiding impulsive decisions that can ultimately stall discussions. Determining the basic feasibility of the relationship from a business perspective should be completed very early in discussions.

The conclusions and recommendations resulting from determining the business needs of the parties will provide a common understanding of the imperatives for alignment and help steer negotiations, particularly as the key deal points for an arrangement become finalized.

Some consideration should be given to the following aspects of alignment:

- How does this arrangement assist the aligned organization's overall vision for the future of how oncology care is delivered in its market?

- Does this arrangement support the hospital's broader physician alignment strategy?

- Will the arrangement facilitate greater clinical coordination and improve efficiency?

Chapter 5

- Are provider needs for competitive compensation and stability addressed?

- Will this arrangement support the community need for oncology services and subspecialty care?

- What should a true partnership involve?

- Are physicians willing and ready to help lead the oncology service line?

- What are "deal breakers" from each party's perspective?

Understand key drivers

The incremental costs associated with hospital/physician alignment often require that parties identify additional revenue streams, either through increased volume or better reimbursement. Financial challenges are particularly significant in oncology-related services because many independent physicians rely on ancillary services for a substantial percentage of their income. (See Figure 5.1 for some potential considerations in the areas of strategy and finance.) In addition, many of these alignment arrangements require large up-front capital expenditures, whether it be to assume the drug inventory of a medical oncology business or to purchase a radiation oncology group's linear accelerators and other related equipment.

To generate new revenue, many hospitals are seeking to convert all or portions of physician practices to provider-based designation. Under provider-based status, physicians receive a reduced Medicare professional fee for selected services, while the employing hospital can bill for overhead expenses. The hospital bills a facility fee to cover the practice costs, which typically exceeds the reduction in

FIGURE 5.1
STRATEGIC AND FINANCIAL CONSIDERATIONS

Strategic	Financial
• Community supply issues • Competitor and community response • Positioning for potential reform changes • Strategic and programmatic growth of key services • Medical staff reactions, particularly independent oncologists • Physician recruitment and retention	• Oncology margin gains (e.g., ancillary and outpatient revenue) • Potential reimbursement changes • Payor reactions • Impact on referral streams • Incremental operating expense (e.g., information technology) requirements • Infrastructure needs

Source: ECG Management Consultants, Inc.

professional fees and can result in a reimbursement advantage, particularly for select oncology services. Even if the Medicare reimbursement differential is insubstantial, the conversion of oncology services to provider-based status can have a considerable commercial reimbursement advantage.

Another approach to enhancing margins is acquiring chemotherapy drugs through the 340B Drug Pricing Program. The 340B program enables participating organizations to purchase qualifying drugs at substantial discounts (an average of 20% to 40% off of retail pricing). If the transaction includes medical oncologists that currently perform infusion therapy services outside the hospital, the parties should conduct a thorough assessment of 340B drug pricing eligibility to identify options

Chapter 5

that maximize the program's benefits. Organizations should at a minimum consider the following questions when evaluating 340B pricing:

- Does the hospital or an affiliated hospital within the system qualify for 340B?

- If the hospital participates in 340B, how large is the practice's chemotherapy program? How many medical oncologists are expected to participate?

- If the hospital participates in 340B, how can it increase its participation through partnerships with community oncologists? And how will the alignment model engage physicians in the program?

- How many qualifying patients (e.g., outpatients, patients with an established relationship with the provider) are expected to participate in the program? What is the expected economic gain?

Ensure proper due diligence

The due diligence process is critical for every transaction and is typically conducted in an iterative fashion, wherein increasingly detailed information is requested from the group. Questions about compensation typically are initiated early in the process. It is critical for the hospital to conduct a thorough assessment of the oncologists' current practice, understanding all revenue streams and expense drivers, before presenting a financial offer to the physicians. This process is important for any specialty acquisition; however, it is particularly important for oncology practices due to the complexities of the practices (e.g., large reliance on ancillary income).

Issues that are commonly identified as a result of the practice assessment include:

- Lack of alignment between compensation and productivity

- Declining compensation and/or productivity over time

- A high level of midlevel services (e.g., infusion management) and/or other services that do not support a work relative value unit (WRVU) compensation model

- High level of outside physician compensation

- Varying compensation plans between employed and shareholder physicians

- Antiquated or poorly maintained capital equipment

- Practices with a large debt load

- Abnormal supply costs relative to production levels

The initial financial review is a critical first step in transaction discussions, but the due diligence process should be ongoing. Due diligence efforts related to implementation planning will begin once a term sheet and/or letter of intent has been finalized. This could include a third-party evaluation of the group's practice (if applicable) and potentially a fair market value (FMV) review of the proposed compensation plan. In addition, there will be a number of other considerations if integrating the group into the hospital (e.g., space planning requirements for provider-based billing compliance). Many of these considerations are outlined in the following sections. To facilitate this process, though, it will be important to share

Chapter 5

the implementation timeline with the physicians so they understand the process as well as the rationale behind what may seem like excessive data requests. Involving one or more of the physicians in the implementation will help ensure that the physician group continues to be educated about the key issues being evaluated.

Development of the Organizational Structure

To ensure successful alignment, the hospital and physicians should jointly develop the governance, management, and operating structures for the new arrangement. Clearly defined organizational structures that delineate the reporting relationships among the physicians and hospital executives are a key element to successfully implementing the intended alignment structure.

Group governance

Governance defines the structure under which the integrated entity sets its strategic direction, manages fiduciary responsibilities, and oversees organizational performance. Specifying organizational authority and accountability is a critical element in the development of a group's culture.

Many top oncology programs elect to establish a governance structure that includes joint representation from physicians and hospital leadership. The balance of membership of these groups will vary depending on the ownership structure and the mix of clinical services and array of physician specialties under the aligned structure. Typically, the governance body will provide oversight for the operations, finances, and planning of the oncology group. Depending on the evolution of the service line, group governance may also be integrated with service line governance structures/functions, as described in Chapter 3. During the planning process, key governance terms should be negotiated and agreed upon, such as:

- Number and selection of governing body members

- Decision-making scope and list of responsibilities

- Role of governing body for the oncology group and (if applicable) within the broader oncology service line

- Voting rights details

- Reserve powers

Management structure

Management of the group should entail experienced administrative leaders to ensure efficient operations but should also incorporate physicians to ensure that they are continuing to monitor operations and are invested in the group's success. In addition, specific management structures should aim to leverage the hospital's employed physician practice capabilities. Defining the management structure in any detail can be a somewhat lengthy process; however, at a minimum, the initial term sheet should outline the following:

- Leadership structure with management relationships noted for key positions

- Job description of key leadership positions

- Appointment of leaders

Chapter 5

Operational and clinical integration

It is also important to develop plans that operationally and clinically integrate the group with the service line in order to meet shared objectives. The decisions that will be required in this design phase include definitions of the following areas:

- Operational and clinical integration across subspecialties
- Branding and marketing activities
- Physician recruiting
- Utilization management
- Information exchange, including use of electronic medical records
- Performance reporting
- Staff employment

Developing a Compensation Plan

Developing a physician compensation methodology that aligns physician incentives with hospital oncology programmatic priorities is critical to ensuring that organizational objectives are achieved. Effective compensation methodologies incorporate variables that encourage clinical productivity, quality and coordination of care, financial stability, and other variables identified by hospital leadership. Several models and key considerations for a compensation plan design are outlined in the following pages.

Key Elements of a Successful Oncology Transaction

Compensation goals and objectives

In designing a compensation plan, it is important to incorporate provisions that support the hospital's broader service line and organizational objectives. Consequently, the first step when designing a compensation plan should be the development of its desired goals and objectives. Ultimately, the goals that are established at the onset of this planning process are used as the evaluation criteria for alternative arrangements. Figure 5.2 outlines common goals.

FIGURE 5.2
COMMON COMPENSATION GOALS

Philosophical	Clinical	Financial	Other Programmatic
• Enhances quality • Aligns compensation with productivity • Is transparent and flexible • Is easy to administer • Is consistent with other hospital payment arrangements	• Improves the patient and physician experience • Promotes coordinated care and clinical integration • Supports subspecialization • Facilitates increased access	• Ensures financial viability • Promotes cost-savings initiatives • Encourages service outreach • Rewards for shared risk	• Supports clinical research efforts • Encourages physician leadership in service line development • Supports other programmatic activity (e.g., citizenship)

Source: ECG Management Consultants, Inc.

Chapter 5

Compensation models

The models in the following discussion represent common physician compensation arrangements. Each model has its advantages and disadvantages. In practice, characteristics from these various models are often combined to create incentives to reward desired behaviors and activities.

Model 1—Income guarantee

- **Structure:** A guaranteed salary regardless of practice productivity or finances, set at a predetermined compensation target. It is typically based on an industry-wide percentile and periodically adjusted to reflect changes in productivity.

- **Advantages:** Stabilizes income, clinical model, and culture for physicians; is easy for hospitals to administer.

- **Disadvantages:** Offers little incentive for increased production and the fewest opportunities to align physician and hospital incentives. May result in diminished productivity. Given oncologists' high income levels, may be difficult to provide a full income guarantee from an FMV perspective. Often associated with high losses in the physician practice.

- **Mitigating considerations:** Minimum work thresholds mitigate productivity risk but can be difficult to negotiate.

- **Risk/potential:** High risk for hospitals; low risk for physicians.

Model 2—Base salary plus production bonus

- **Structure:** A guaranteed salary supplemented by a bonus based on WRVUs, new patient visits, and so forth, beyond a set threshold. The bonus may be based on individual productivity, total group productivity in certain situations, or a combination of both.

- **Advantages:** Potentially increases physician income; aligns financial incentives with hospital.

- **Disadvantages:** Offers less income stability for physicians and no incentive for nonclinical physician activities such as administrative contributions to the oncology service line. Oncology ancillary income streams (e.g., infusion) do not necessarily correlate to a WRVU model.

- **Mitigating considerations:** Model could incorporate additional incentives for nonclinical work. The threshold should be set low enough so the production bonus is a significant portion of total compensation.

- **Risk/potential:** Moderate risk/moderate upside potential for physicians depending on where the threshold is set.

Model 3—Base salary plus multiple bonuses

- **Structure:** A guaranteed salary supplemented by bonuses based on factors such as productivity, quality and outcomes, outreach and referral relationships, program development, and patient satisfaction.

Chapter 5

- **Advantages:** Flexibly aligns incentives for nonclinical activities. May better align compensation to physicians' historical income levels. Aspects such as standardizing clinical practices may be self-funding.

- **Disadvantages:** Developing service line metrics and valuing nonclinical work can be difficult. May weaken the direct link between compensation and production.

- **Mitigating considerations:** Time studies could be utilized to set payments. WRVUs or other productivity metrics could also be included in the formula. Funding mechanisms for bonus pools need to be determined.

- **Risk/potential:** Moderate risk/moderate-to-high upside potential for physicians.

Model 4—Pure productivity

- **Structure:** No salary guarantee. Physicians are compensated at a fixed rate per WRVU, patient visit, etc., either individually or as a group. The compensation rate may increase for production above certain thresholds.

- **Advantages:** Ensures hospital costs are in line with productivity; is the typical model for professional service agreements, and more prevalent in employment.

- **Disadvantages:** Offers limited income stability for physicians and does not align incentives for physician participation in nonclinical service line work unless these components are added.

- **Mitigating considerations:** Model could incorporate additional incentives for nonclinical work.

- **Risk/potential:** Moderate risk/moderate-to-high upside potential.

Unique considerations

In addition to the general compensation provisions of an agreement, there are unique considerations that emerge in various transaction discussions depending on the dynamics of a particular practice.

Aggregate versus individual payment methodologies

Physician compensation can be based on a pool or allocated individually, depending in particular on the culture of the group. Pooled compensation is often most applicable in professional services agreements (particularly because organizations often receive payment in aggregate and use different allocation methodologies for their individual physician compensation); however, it can also apply to employed arrangements for practices that utilize an equal shares model and believe strongly that a pooled methodology creates a collegial, collaborative group culture. Within groups where there is disparity in production, a model that creates both shared and individual incentives may be more appropriate. Pooled compensation models should have the appropriate controls to manage total compensation at FMV levels.

Infusion suite services

For medical oncology practices that heavily use midlevel providers for the management of infusion services, it is important to consider how productivity and expense will impact their compensation model. In particular, the reporting of physician

Chapter 5

productivity through WRVUS will be impacted, as physicians will no longer receive credit for this production if infusion services are transitioned to a hospital-based billing model (because infusion therapy is a designated health service). Depending on the magnitude of this activity, it may be important to structure an arrangement that allows for physicians' continued management of infusion services.

Increasingly, hospitals are opting to create agreements that compensate physicians for management of the infusion suite. Several options are available, depending on the particulars of an arrangement. Many opt for a fixed fee stipend that compensates physicians for services related to infusion suite management. Others incorporate a payment per WRVU premium that reflects incremental compensation associated with management services. An alternate but similar approach to this last methodology is the incorporation of a WRVU credit for clinical services that correlates to infusion management activity. Regardless of the approach, hospitals will need to be cautious in developing their preferred methodology to ensure that payment is in no way tied to hospital-based volume growth.

Service incentives

Hospitals generally recognize that production-driven plans will need to evolve to reflect changing practice patterns and economics, but there is a reluctance to get too far ahead of reimbursement changes. Production-based compensation plans (typically measured in WRVUs) continue to be the favored methodology for hospitals, and they often utilize productivity tiers that disproportionately reward high producers and provide strong incentives at the margin. These plans reflect the current economics of physician payment, which is still based almost entirely on clinical work measures.

Key Elements of a Successful Oncology Transaction

Although hospitals typically incorporate some type of performance or quality bonus into their compensation models, the measures are often not based on stretch goals because defining, valuing, tracking, and measuring outcomes can prove difficult. They can provide a huge boon to executing service line strategies, though, and more institutions are starting to incorporate these incentives and make them a larger portion of total compensation (see Figure 5.3 for examples).

FIGURE 5.3
COMMON SERVICE INCENTIVE BONUS STRUCTURES

Category	Examples
Quality	• Amercian College of Surgeons quality indicators • American College of Radiology-American Society for Therapeutic Radiology and Oncology accreditation • Reporting of select Physician Quality Reporting System variables • Participation in multidisciplinary clinics • Adherence to established clinical pathways • Standardization of drug regimens and purchasing
Operations	• Standardization of clinical processes and/or forms • Improvements in select operational metrics
Patient satisfaction	• Survey participation and achievement (e.g., Press Ganey Associates, Inc.) • Availability of appointments
Service line involvement	• Participation in tumor boards • Development of continuing medical education programs • Outreach visits to referring physicians • Participation in hospital leadership roles
Financial	• Clinical market share • Cost-savings bonuses • Device or supply standardization

Source: ECG Management Consultants, Inc.

Chapter 5

Key questions to address when evaluating service incentives include:

- **Picking stretch targets:** Are the metrics attainable? How much effort will be required to reach targets? How should targets be adjusted year over year?

- **Physician control:** Are the metrics related to initiatives under the control of the oncologists? Is there a balance of metrics related to each subspecialty?

- **Areas of emphasis:** How should each metric be weighted (e.g., equally, by importance, by level of difficulty, by time commitment)?

- **Performance measurement:** How easily can the proposed service incentives be tracked and/or measured? Who will be responsible for managing this program?

- **Alignment of goals of hospital and group:** Are the metrics encouraging both the desired group behavior and meeting service line goals?

- **Process-related metrics:** How can we balance metrics aimed at developing processes versus attaining specific measurable levels of achievement?

- **Periodic review:** How often should the planning objectives be reviewed by the hospital and the physicians?

Use of service incentives in physician compensation models is an emerging trend that will continue to grow, particularly in light of ongoing healthcare reform efforts that emphasize patient outcomes and episode-based care.

Surgical oncology call coverage restrictions

With increasing subspecialization of surgical oncologists, many physicians are no longer clinically able or personally willing to cover general surgery call. If the hospital's current emergency department (ED) call coverage arrangement or medical staff bylaws require the physicians to take call, the transaction may require additional funding to compensate surgeons to take general calls.

Other nonclinical duties

Depending on the scope of a particular agreement, other nonclinical duties may need to be taken into account, including but not limited to the following:

- Practice management responsibilities
- Outreach staffing
- Medical directorships and other hospital responsibilities
- Clinical research

Frequently, these types of services are incorporated into the compensation agreement through various performance-related bonuses; some activities (e.g., medical directorships) may reflect separate agreements.

Practice acquisition

If applicable to the arrangement, practice acquisition details should be defined early in the planning process. Hospitals typically purchase a practice's hard assets at FMV. When engaging in the acquisition process, parties should consider the following:

Chapter 5

- **Timing:** One of the most common causes for delay in transaction discussions, particularly for large group acquisitions, is the valuation. Consequently, it is helpful to initiate a practice valuation early in the planning process, potentially once a term sheet has been finalized and/or a letter of intent has been signed.

- **Valuation firm selection:** The most successful valuation process usually relies on one third-party valuation firm to conduct the analysis. To ensure trust in the analysis, it is important to have buy-in from each party in valuation firm selection. Some organizations opt to each hire its respective valuation firm to conduct separate analyses; however, this process can often be cumbersome and has the potential to significantly delay the transaction process as the parties reconcile the two reports.

- **Tangible versus intangible assets:** In recent years, most transactions have excluded goodwill and focused solely on tangible/hard assets. Increasingly, some hospitals do value select intangibles (e.g., medical records, workforce in place), but the inclusion of intangibles often only applies to large group acquisitions.

- **Stock versus asset sale:** When acquiring a practice, parties have the option of utilizing two different types of sales—an asset sale and a stock sale. In an asset sale, the hospital is purchasing a defined list of assets and assumes a defined list of liabilities; consequently, the liability of unknown future claims against the corporation is retained by the physicians. This is the most common method used in practice acquisitions. In contrast, under a stock sale, the hospital assumes the liability for all unknown future claims.

Physicians are increasingly requesting the latter option; however, it is important to note that, with the addition of these liabilities, the physician stock is worth less to the hospital than the known quantities of assets and liabilities in an asset sale. In addition, if a stock sale is ultimately considered, there are several steps that should be taken to limit future liabilities. For example, the hospital could retain a portion of sale proceeds or insure against future claims.

- **Equipment leases:** The disposition of the oncology office often depends on whether it is owned by the practice or the office is located in leased space. In addition, oncologists may have engaged in various other lease arrangements that could impact the valuation price. Because the assignment of the various assets to the hospital is usually a condition of closing, any last-minute, unforeseen expenses typically result in incremental costs to the hospital that were previously not budgeted. Consequently, it is important to engage in a due diligence process early on that identifies all relevant agreements and associated costs for the practice.

Key terms
Contract term

Although most oncology agreements are structured for a term of two to three years, an increasing number of organizations are opting for longer contract terms (e.g., five years). Physicians prefer the financial stability associated with a longer contract, and hospitals often consider it part of their broader retention strategy by incorporating vesting provisions into the agreement. For example, some organizations withhold a portion of the physician bonus for a predetermined vesting period;

only after completing the predetermined term would physicians be eligible to receive 100% of their bonus compensation. Due to unforeseen environmental changes, longer contract terms offer some level of additional hospital risk; consequently, it is important to incorporate reset provisions into the compensation plan that ensure some payment flexibility in relation to market changes. Organizations should ensure that any FMV assessment of an alignment arrangement covers the term of the agreement; longer-term arrangements could require periodic FMV updates.

Agreement renewal
Regardless of the contract length, most agreements include a periodic reset every few years to ensure that physician compensation remains commensurate with the FMV. Organizations utilize a variety of industry benchmarks, preferring those with a wide circulation and large sample size.

Some contracts do utilize a fixed payment mechanism in the compensation plan for a predefined period of time (e.g., a five-year compensation per WRVU rate); in these cases, it is still important to incorporate explicit provisions to ensure market-level compensation and FMV compliance. Typically, this involves the utilization of a payment corridor that limits the upside compensation (e.g., 90th percentile or includes events that would trigger an FMV in mid-term) and adjusts for diminished productivity (e.g., a 15% reduction in the compensation rate for a 15% drop in WRVU productivity).

Noncompete agreements
Noncompete provisions generally restrict physicians from competing within a predefined geographic area for one to two years. Restrictions range in complexity

but generally limit physicians' ability to perform specialty services in competing hospitals/facilities within the employer's primary, secondary, and/or tertiary service areas. In situations where the hospital acquires a physician practice, the noncompete may also include provisions that require physicians to pay back a prorated portion of the practice acquisition costs if they terminate the agreement within a predetermined time frame (e.g., two years from the date of employment). However, hospitals should resist the temptation to overreach in writing a noncompete agreement. In many states, if a judge finds that the time or geographic restrictions are unreasonable to protect the hospital's legitimate economic interests, the entire agreement may be void and unenforceable.

Implementation

The key to a long-term successful transaction is effective alignment and integration into a coordinated service line that is capable of achieving the parties' intended goals. It is at the implementation phase immediately following closing that many well-conceived transactions fail. Although often overlooked in the haste of events that typically precede the closing, it is critical that the hospital and physicians carefully plan and execute the implementation steps, which is frequently a two-phase process.

Phase I: Plan development
Following the signing of a term sheet, the parties should develop detailed plans for implementation and integration, including:

Chapter 5

- Identifying key stakeholders and knowledge experts from the respective organizations. This typically includes practice administrators and staff from the physician groups.

- Creating an implementation plan (see sidebar for more information).

- Communicating the implementation plan to work groups and seeking input on potential plan changes.

Phase II: Plan implementation

Upon closing, hospital leadership will need to implement this proposed plan by engaging in the following:

- Creating a project manager or project management team to oversee implementation

    - This may encompass several work groups depending on the size and complexity of the implementation

    - In certain circumstances, using independent, external resources to advise or lead implementation through a project management office may better serve the combined entity because it can overcome institutional biases on either side to make decisions that are in its best interests

- Reporting results, progress, and risks to leadership to expedite decision-making and the implementation of risk-mitigation plans

- Continuing to identify cross-functional dependencies

Key Elements of a Successful Oncology Transaction

- Monitoring key issues to ensure resolution

- Providing interim management where necessary until permanent candidates can be hired

A well thought out, detailed implementation plan is required to transition responsibilities to the new structure without impairing business performance, employee morale, or patient service. In particular, the hospital needs to take special steps to ensure it makes sound operational decisions and proactively communicates with the physicians. Issues will arise, and maintaining open communication through regularly scheduled leadership meetings and weekly implementation updates is critical to managing the change.

DEVELOPING AN IMPLEMENTATION PLAN

The details of an implementation plan will vary based on the alignment model and the characteristics of the respective organizations. Key features of the implementation plan typically include:

- Identifying, measuring, and monitoring key activities and critical success factors

- Defining target dates for completion and specifying major milestones (e.g., 30-, 60-, and 90-day accomplishments)

- Identifying dependencies among tasks to properly sequence work

- Highlighting difficult integration issues and decisions that warrant board approval

- Identifying milestones and accomplishments

- Assigning accountability of each task to an individual who will be responsible for ensuring that work is completed on time

Chapter 5

Key Takeaways

Properly structured, economic oncology alignment arrangements can be mutually beneficial to both parties. The most successful transactions typically apply the following approach:

- Using a rigorous, disciplined, and timely process when negotiating term sheet decisions

    - Initiating key tasks (e.g., practice valuation process) early in transaction discussions to set parameters

    - Understanding market risks and trends before engaging in detailed compensation discussions

- Proactively establishing a shared vision and set of goals that define success

- Determining an appropriate vehicle to meet current and future service line needs

    - Incorporating terms that are tailored to the group by leveraging their strengths and addressing their weaknesses

    - Creating incentives within the compensation plan to align physicians with the hospital's organizational priorities

    - Developing a structure that encourages and allows for strong physician leadership in service line planning and management

- Creating a long-term, financially viable relationship

- Determining an appropriate billing designation to maximize reimbursement opportunities

- Assessing 340B cost-savings opportunities

• Preparing and executing a thorough, detailed implementation plan to ensure effective physician integration upon the transaction's close

CHAPTER 6

Navigating the Challenges of Oncology Reimbursement

Although all healthcare specialties are facing pressure on reimbursement, oncology is an especially complex and economically challenging service. Cancer care is expensive and politically sensitive, with doctors, hospitals, drug companies, legislators, and insurance companies all having major roles in the evolution of how services are delivered and paid for. To understand the economic realities of oncology programs, the basic points that should be remembered include the following:

- The demand for oncology services is growing

- Oncology care is predominantly provided on an outpatient basis

- Medicare is the major payer for oncology services

- Infusion services and drugs are the main source of revenue in medical oncology

- Technical reimbursement drives profit margins in radiation oncology

Not surprisingly, healthcare policy deliberations have had a major impact on oncology, including several provisions in the 2010 Patient Protection and Affordable Care Act that emphasize lowering expenditures while enhancing

Chapter 6

coordination and integration of cancer care. Seven of the top 10 Medicare Part B drugs are used to treat either cancer or the side effects associated with chemotherapy.[1] Medicare spending and drug utilization were also front and center during the 2011 debt ceiling negotiations between the White House and Congress—with lawmakers at one point calling for cuts of up to $3 billion for cancer drugs. While less draconian measures were adopted, it is clear that both political and market forces are at work to change oncology reimbursement in the coming years.

These financial pressures have begun to change the organizational relationships between physicians, hospitals, and, in many ways, patients, as noted in other chapters of this book. More oncology physicians are choosing to move their drug infusion business from their private practices to hospital-based infusion suites. This momentum will likely increase as reimbursement pressures continue to mount. New contractual arrangements are being conceived between medical oncologists and their hospital partners to continue the supervision and coordination of patient care in the hospital environment.

This chapter will provide the background and historical context necessary to understand how oncology services are paid for, what changes in reimbursement are possible or likely, and what the economic and organizational implications of those changes will be. This discussion will include why oncology represents a major opportunity for hospitals to provide leadership in integrating the currently fragmented providers of cancer care.

> **BREAKING NEWS: DRUG SHORTAGES**
>
> The increasing and disconcerting trend of drug shortages, including those used in the treatment of cancer, is one manifestation of the challenges of drug reimbursement. In August 2011, *The New York Times* reported that at least 180 drugs crucial in the treatment of childhood leukemia, breast and colon cancer, infections, and other diseases were declared to be in short supply in the first half of the year alone—the most ever.[2] And forecasts suggest that the trend of drug shortages will continue at least into the near future.
>
> The shortage of drugs not only has a significant impact on care, but it also puts additional pressures on drug prices, often resulting in acquisition costs that can far exceed reimbursement levels. Evidenced by the emergence of parallel or "gray" market vendors in the supply chain for these drugs, the markup (particularly for those drugs used to treat the critically ill) can be astounding. According to a study published by Premier, the group purchasing cooperative, the average markup for 1,745 gray-market offers to providers for these drugs was 650%, and even higher for some critical care drugs. In fact, three drugs used in the treatment of cancer (cytarabine, dexamethasone, and leucovorin) ranked at the very top; in some cases, these drugs had markups approaching 4,000%.[3]

Keys to Oncology Reimbursement: Legislation, Drugs, Professional Fees

Legislative impact

Each round of healthcare-related legislation aims to reduce expenditures, whether by reducing utilization or lowering per unit reimbursement. The past several years have seen a renewed focus on oncology costs as the payment methodology for drugs was redefined and imaging services were bundled. Figure 6.1 provides a summary of the key legislation and associated implications.

Chapter 6

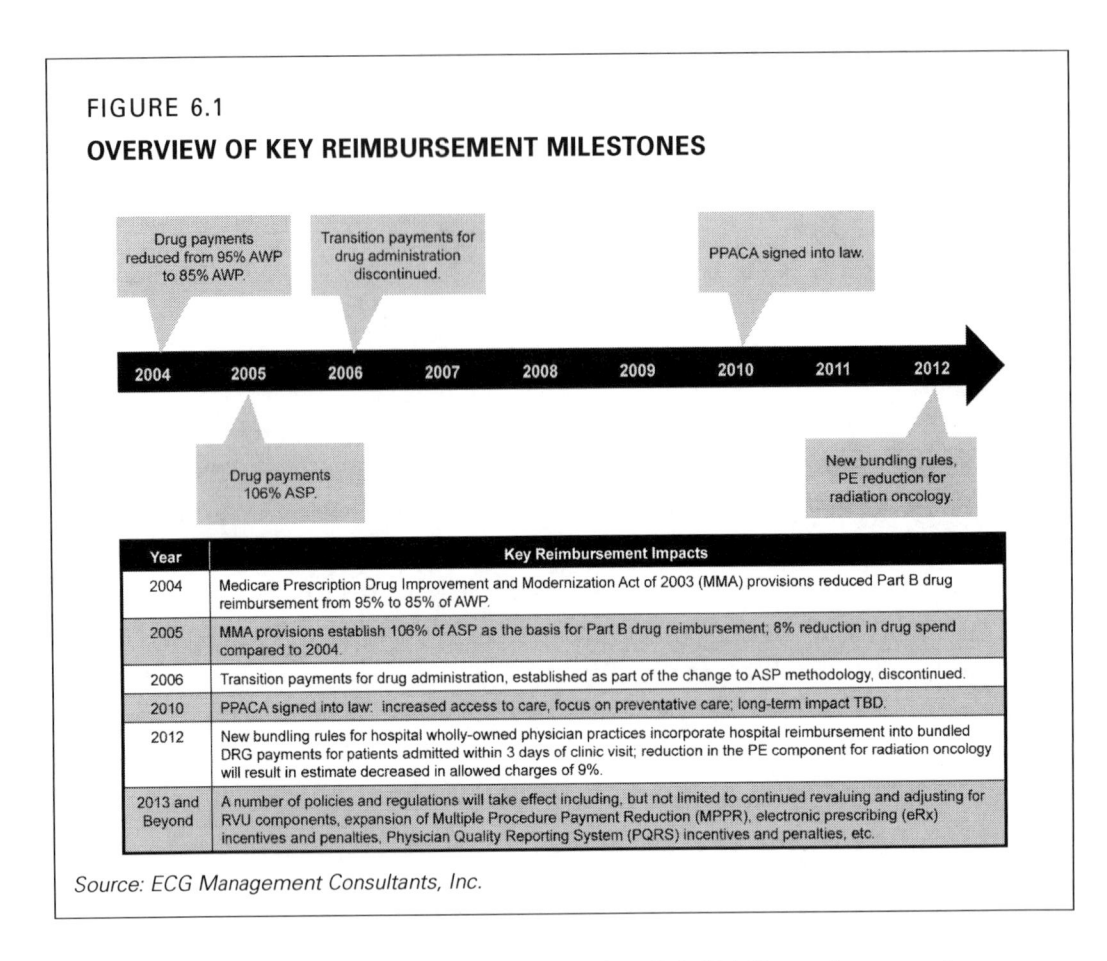

FIGURE 6.1
OVERVIEW OF KEY REIMBURSEMENT MILESTONES

Timeline (2004–2012):
- 2004: Drug payments reduced from 95% AWP to 85% AWP.
- 2005: Drug payments 106% ASP.
- 2006: Transition payments for drug administration discontinued.
- 2010: PPACA signed into law.
- 2012: New bundling rules, PE reduction for radiation oncology.

Year	Key Reimbursement Impacts
2004	Medicare Prescription Drug Improvement and Modernization Act of 2003 (MMA) provisions reduced Part B drug reimbursement from 95% to 85% of AWP.
2005	MMA provisions establish 106% of ASP as the basis for Part B drug reimbursement; 8% reduction in drug spend compared to 2004.
2006	Transition payments for drug administration, established as part of the change to ASP methodology, discontinued.
2010	PPACA signed into law: increased access to care, focus on preventative care; long-term impact TBD.
2012	New bundling rules for hospital wholly-owned physician practices incorporate hospital reimbursement into bundled DRG payments for patients admitted within 3 days of clinic visit; reduction in the PE component for radiation oncology will result in estimate decreased in allowed charges of 9%.
2013 and Beyond	A number of policies and regulations will take effect including, but not limited to continued revaluing and adjusting for RVU components, expansion of Multiple Procedure Payment Reduction (MPPR), electronic prescribing (eRx) incentives and penalties, Physician Quality Reporting System (PQRS) incentives and penalties, etc.

Source: ECG Management Consultants, Inc.

The Medicare Payment Advisory Commission (MedPAC) continues to cite expenses related to ancillary services (particularly diagnostic imaging) and drugs as a primary focus and driver of healthcare expenditures. In both 2006 and 2007, the commission published reports on the effects of drug payment policies on oncology and other specialties. In addition, in its 2011 report to Congress, the commission explicitly stated its concern regarding "the expansion of physician investment in imaging, other diagnostic tests, and therapeutic services (e.g., physical therapy, radiation therapy) and the potential for self-referral to lead to higher volume." The report goes on to note that MedPAC intends to revisit options in the future to narrow the Stark Law exceptions related to these services provided in the physician office setting.

> **PROJECTION**
>
> Based on the continued policy discussions surrounding imaging and drug costs, there will be continued downward pressure on reimbursement related to these services, which will be the clear trend for the foreseeable future.

Drug reimbursement: Driving alignment

Most medical oncology practice revenues and profitability are derived from the drug infusion services provided by physicians. In fact, in many cases the revenue related to these services can top 90% of all revenue.[4] For many years, Medicare, followed by private payers, has attempted to reduce the spread between what doctors pay for oncology drugs and what Medicare pays them for those drugs when they are administered to a patient. In order to fully comprehend the trends in drug reimbursement and understand an oncologist's point of view, one must appreciate the history of drug reimbursement changes over the last several years.

Prior to 2005, Medicare drug prices were based on the average wholesale price (AWP) and reimbursed based on a percentage of this number. AWP was essentially the retail price of the drug based on data from drug manufacturers, distributors, and other suppliers. While most drug purchasing contracts are confidential, it was generally accepted that the AWP of drugs grossly overstated the actual market

Chapter 6

prices. Medicare attempted to remedy this problem by reimbursing providers based on a percentage less than the listed AWP (and to date, many commercial payers have followed suit). However, despite a greater than 10% reduction in the drug payment factor, reimbursement for physician-administered drugs remained much higher than acquisition costs. Between 1997 and 2003, spending on Part B drugs increased at an average rate of 25% per year. Therefore, in 2005, Medicare set payments for drugs based on a new methodology called average sales price (ASP) (see Figure 6.2).

FIGURE 6.2
IMPACT OF MEDICARE PART B DRUG PRICING/REIMBURSEMENT*

Year	Reimbursement Policy	Estimated Payments (in billions of dollars)	Percentage Change
2004	85% of AWP	$3.38	Transition to ASP
2005	106% of ASP	$2.90	14% decrease in payments

*Analysis based on all 2004 Medicare claims submissions identified as "Hematology/Oncology." Estimated payments reflect 2004 Current Procedural Terminology code volume for codes identified as "Other Drugs" or "Chemotherapy" based on the Berenson-Eggers Type of Service definition and 2004 and 2005 Medicare Part B drug payment limits published by the Centers for Medicare & Medicaid Services.

Source: ECG Management Consultants, Inc.

The ASP methodology attempts to determine the actual market price for drugs based on sales data provided by manufacturers on a quarterly basis. This data is the net of price concessions and rebates and is limited to sales in the United States. ASP is set prospectively based on the prices from the previous two quarters.

Today, Medicare reimbursement for drugs in an oncology private practice is 106% of ASP. Extra transition payments for infusion administration were extended until 2006 and then ended. As anticipated, the ASP payment methodology has reduced the margins generated from drugs within an oncology practice. And while there is some controversy regarding the inclusion of prompt payment and other discounts in the calculation of ASP, it has been found that most drugs can be purchased at rates lower than Medicare reimbursement levels.

Centers for Medicare & Medicaid Services (CMS) data illustrate that in 2005 (see Figure 6.3), after it moved to the ASP methodology, its spending on Part B drugs declined 8%.[5] In 2006, MedPAC released a congressional report on the impact of adjustments to oncology payments. The study estimated that physicians provided 13% more chemotherapy infusion sessions in 2005 than in 2004.[6] However, the same study showed that Medicare paid 14% less for chemotherapy drugs during this time under the new payment methodology. Given the tangible cost savings, with no indication of a reduction in quality or level of patient care, CMS has continued to focus on reducing drug spending as a means to curb Medicare spending.

Chapter 6

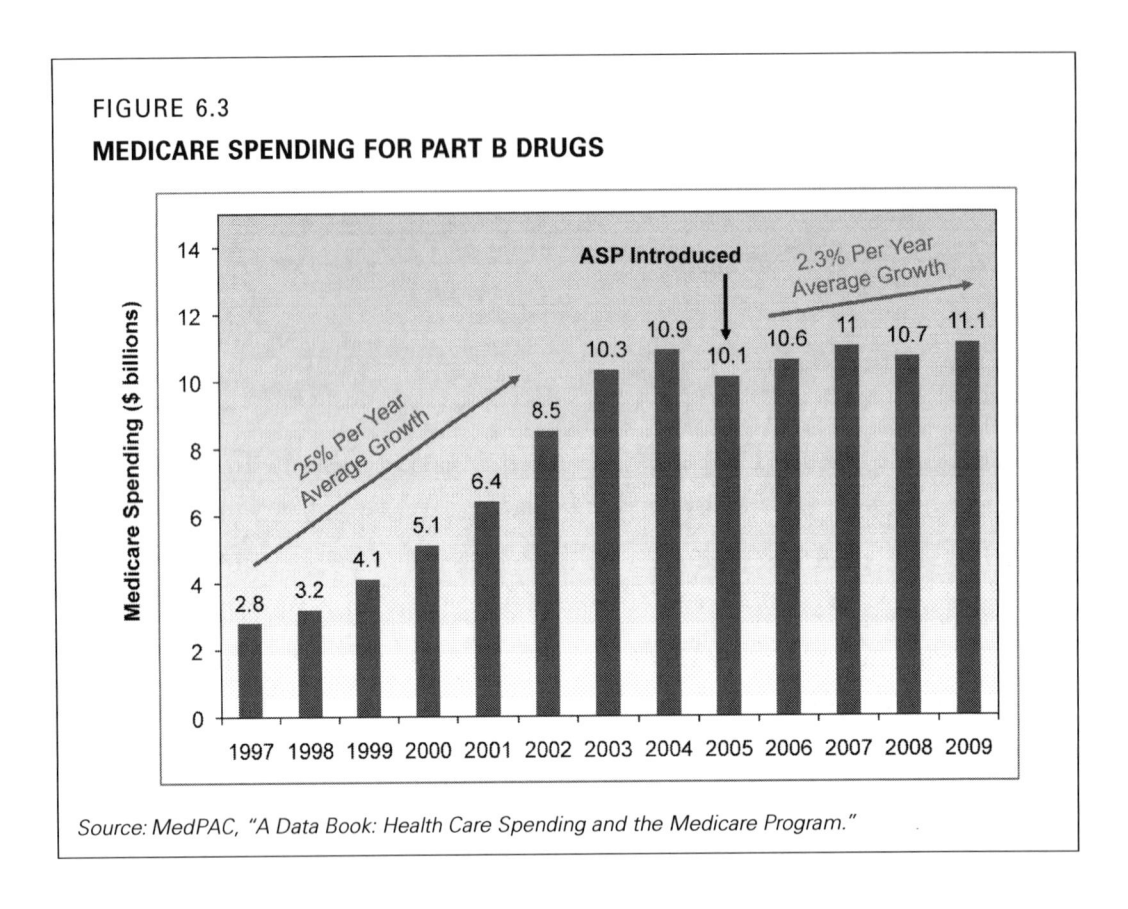

FIGURE 6.3
MEDICARE SPENDING FOR PART B DRUGS

Year	Medicare Spending ($ billions)
1997	2.8
1998	3.2
1999	4.1
2000	5.1
2001	6.4
2002	8.5
2003	10.3
2004	10.9
2005	10.1
2006	10.6
2007	11
2008	10.7
2009	11.1

25% Per Year Average Growth (1997–2004)
ASP Introduced (2005)
2.3% Per Year Average Growth (2005–2009)

Source: MedPAC, "A Data Book: Health Care Spending and the Medicare Program."

In 2011, CMS has proposed yet another change under which it would substitute average manufacturer price (AMP) or widely available market price for ASP in order to bring reimbursement levels even closer to actual acquisition costs for certain drugs. CMS has suggested specifically limiting the substitution of 103% of AMP for 106% of ASP, including the following:

- When ASP exceeds AMP by 5% or more for two consecutive quarters or three of the four prior quarters

- Only when the comparison provided by the Office of Inspector General is based on the same set of National Drug Codes

Oncology practices have responded to this downward pressure on reimbursement by increasing the operational efficiency of their practices (again, drugs can comprise upwards of 90% percent of all revenue in some cases). In fact, in both 2006 and 2007, when studying the impact of the changes in drug reimbursement methodology, MedPAC noted that "physicians responded to the changes by cutting costs and increasing efficiency (particularly with respect to drug purchasing activities), finding new sources of revenue (e.g., imaging), and selecting more profitable patients."[7]

TWO TIERS OF CANCER TREATMENT

In many areas of the country, uninsured and underinsured patients (without supplemental insurance) are often sent to nonprofit hospital infusion centers for treatment because a private practice is at risk for the high cost of chemotherapy. This trend raises several issues in terms of patient access, costs to the healthcare system, and potentially quality.

- **Patient access:** In the future, access to specific treatments, clinical research, and physician specialists may be limited by location. Patients may be required to seek treatment far from home.

- **Cost:** MedPAC estimated that 9% of all beneficiaries have no source of supplemental coverage, putting an increasing burden on safety net hospitals for these services.

- **Quality of care:** While the physician may continue to manage the patient's care, access to hospital data must be seamless to appropriately adjust and respond to changes with the patient. Electronic health records are becoming more common; however, access to specialty data such as oncology treatment planning is complex and not well coordinated at a community level.

National and local entities have expressed concerns about these trends. However, to date, there have been no long-term proposals for solutions to this issue.

Chapter 6

> **PROJECTION**
>
> Today, most practices have maximized operational efficiency. As reductions in drug reimbursement continue, it is likely that independent oncologists' income will erode, increasing their interest in seeking employment or other affiliation with hospitals.

Private practice reimbursement

Although there will continue to be downward pressure on professional fees, these changes will not impact medical oncology and radiation oncology in the same manner. The remainder of this section describes how some of the trends previously noted specifically affect these subspecialties separately.

Medical oncology

Physician practices rely on Medicare Part B reimbursement for evaluation and management (E&M) codes, infusion administration, and drug charges. The continued changes to relative value units (RVU) and multiple procedure payment reduction (MPPR) policy are not predicted to have any significant impact on hematology/oncology from 2011 to 2012. According to CMS' Calendar Year 2012 Physician Fee Schedule Proposed Rule, the estimated total impact of these changes on RVUs is 0.0% in 2012 and -2% in 2013. However, the Relative Value Update Committee (RUC)[8] is currently studying three chemotherapy current procedural terminology (CPT) codes that have not been reviewed in more than six years for potential revaluing (see Figure 6.4).

FIGURE 6.4
RUC REVALUING INTIATIVE: MEDICAL ONCOLOGY CODES

CPT Code	Description
96365	Intravenous infusion, for therapy, prophylaxis, or diagnosis up to 1 hour
96367	Tx/Proph/Diag, additional sequential infusion up to 1 hour
96413	Chemotherapy admin, IV infusion, up to 1 hour

Source: ECG Management Consultants, Inc.

Despite the adjustments being made to RVU calculations and select codes, the changes in drug reimbursement methodology have been the major impact on reimbursement for private practice medical oncology.

As shown in Figure 6.5, 84% of Medicare payments to oncologists were for Part B drugs and drug administration (72% and 12%, respectively) while only 12% were for E&M services.[9] Although medical oncology revenue continues to be heavily weighted toward drugs and drug administration, the margin on these services has dramatically declined over the years. In fact, according to data recently published in the American Society of Clinical Oncology's *Journal of Oncology Practice*, the average drug margin in 2009 was 8% of total revenue,[10] down from margins as high as 45% as recently as 2002.

Chapter 6

FIGURE 6.5
MEDICARE PAYMENTS TO ONCOLOGISTS BY TYPE OF SERVICE

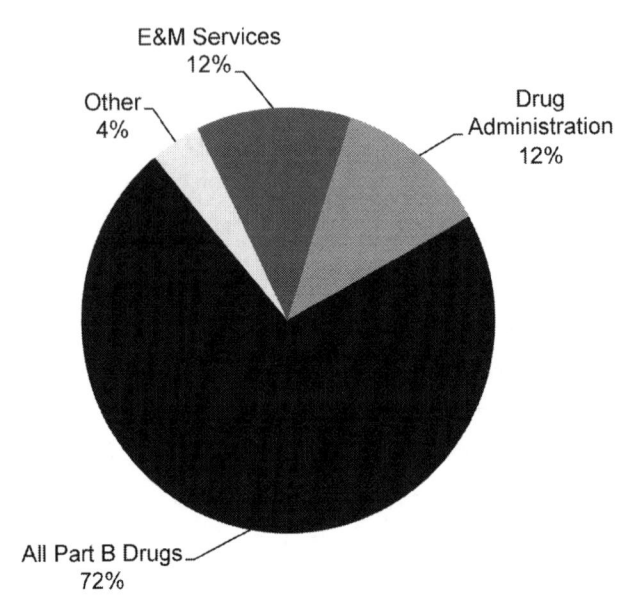

- E&M Services 12%
- Drug Administration 12%
- Other 4%
- All Part B Drugs 72%

Source: MedPAC, "Report to the Congress, Effects of Medicare Payment Changes on Oncology Services," January 2006.

Recent data from the Medical Group Management Association supports these projections, indicating that private medical oncology practices have seen a significant decline in professional fee collections and compensation. Between 2008 and 2010, the median physician collections for professional charges declined almost 30% (see Figure 6.6).

Navigating the Challenges of Oncology Reimbursement

FIGURE 6.6
PHYSICIAN COLLECTIONS FOR PROFESSIONAL CHARGES 2008–2010*

Year	Median	Percentage Change From Previous Year
2010	$486,293	–9.0%
2009	$534,573	–22.8%
2008	$692,879	N/A

*2008 to 2010 Medical Group Management Association *Physician Production and Compensation Surveys*, Table 5.6 Physician Collections for Professional Charges (TC/NPP Excluded) by Hospital Ownership–Hematology/Oncology.

This likely reflects both reductions in reimbursement levels as well as a number of practices shifting infusion services into the hospital setting. Meanwhile, median compensation levels for private medical oncology physicians remained relatively flat (see Figure 6.7), increasing only 3% during this time period, while hospital-employed medical oncologists saw median compensation levels increase almost 11% (although median compensation levels remain slightly lower for employed physicians, that gap is narrowing quickly).

PROJECTION

Declines in private oncologists' revenue, combined with increasingly competitive financial arrangements with hospitals, will drive many medical oncologists toward aligning with hospitals. This represents a major opportunity for hospitals that are interested in establishing an integrated oncology service line.

Chapter 6

FIGURE 6.7
PHYSICIAN COMPENSATION (HEMATOLOGY/ONCOLOGY) 2008–2010*

	Hospital-Owned		Not Hospital-Owned	
Year	Median	Percentage Change From Previous Year	Median	Percentage Change From Previous Year
2010	$375,000	18.1%	$404,412	0.8%
2009	$317,543	−6.3%	$401,125	2.5%
2008	$338,854	N/A	$391,203	N/A

*2008 to 2010 Medical Group Management Association *Physician Production and Compensation Surveys*, Table 1.6 Physician Compensation (More Than 1 Year in Specialty) by Hospital Ownership—Hematology/Oncology.

THE FUTURE: ORAL DRUGS

The rise of oral forms of chemotherapy present an interesting dynamic to the overall reimbursement landscape for private practice medical oncology physicians. While the lifestyle benefits for some patients are obvious (particularly as patients are living longer and require treatment and supportive care agents for longer periods of time), physicians are not reimbursed for oral administration.

Unlike traditional chemotherapy infusion, where physicians are reimbursed for both the cost and administration of the drug, physicians write prescriptions for oral medications that are then filled at a pharmacy. Because physicians are not incurring the cost of the medication (pharmacies are) and patients administer the drug themselves, physicians receive no revenue for patients treated with only oral medications. In this circumstance (and under current reimbursement rules), the only real opportunity for physicians to realize revenue from oral treatments is by directly dispensing the medication from the practice location. As the efficacy and demand for these drugs increase, more medical oncology practices may seek to offer dispensing services directly to their patients.

Radiation oncology

For radiation oncology, it is technology rather than drugs that plays a significant role in the reimbursement landscape. The past few years have seen the emergence of new treatment technologies such as intensity-modulated radiation therapy (IMRT), image-guided radiation therapy, and stereotactic body radiation therapy, all of which garner higher Medicare reimbursement than more traditional forms of radiation therapy. In fact, the vast majority of practices across the United States employ at least one of these techniques, which is why these practices have seen a substantial increase in total reimbursement over the past few years.

Nevertheless, downward pressures on reimbursement are also a major factor in radiation oncology. The 2005 Deficit Reduction Act imposed caps on certain imaging services, such as MRI and PET/CT scans, that are used in conjunction with radiation therapy. In 2010, radiation oncology centers were given a reprieve from CMS' proposed cuts to the service—instead of a 19% reduction, CMS decided to implement a 5% reduction, phased in over a four-year period. As a result, freestanding radiation oncology centers will continue to be targeted in 2012 and 2013 as part of continued changes to RVUs, specifically the transition to a new practice expense (PE) value component. IMRT (CPT 77418), initially reimbursed at very high levels as a new treatment modality, has experienced a decline in payment levels over the course of the past few years.

The RUC is also studying three potentially "misvalued" radiation oncology CPT codes (see Figure 6.8).

Chapter 6

FIGURE 6.8

RUC REVALUING INITIATIVE: RADIATION CODES

CPT Code	Description
77421	Stereoscopic x-ray guidance
77301	Radiotherapy dose plan, IMRT
77014	CT scan for therapy guide

Source: ECG Management Consultants, Inc.

CMS is considering expanding the MPPR, which may have a direct impact on oncology imaging services moving forward. Although no specific rule has been proposed at this time, the following three options are currently subject for comment:

- Apply the MPPR to the technical component of all imaging codes (not just advanced imaging)

- Apply the MPPR to the professional component of all imaging codes

- Apply the MPPR to the technical component of all diagnostic codes

Applying the MPPR to the technical component of all diagnostic codes will negatively affect radiation oncology and radiology. In CMS' Calendar Year 2012 PFS Proposed Rule, both the application of MPPR and the decrease in the radiation oncology PE weight will result in an approximately 6% decrease in allowed charges for radiation therapy centers in 2012. Without the transition period, the full impact to radiation therapy centers was projected to be a 10% decrease.[11] Even if certain provisions are changed when the rule is finalized, the consistent theme of decreasing reimbursement will continue for freestanding radiation oncology centers.

Implications for Hospitals

The implementation of reimbursement policies mentioned in the previous section is clearly driving change for the local oncologist private practice model. Hospitals, at least in the short-term, are able to fare better from a total reimbursement standpoint in these circumstances because of reimbursement advantages related to enhance contracts for particular services (e.g., radiation therapy, diagnostic imaging, infusions), provider-based status, and 340B drug pricing for those who qualify. Each of these areas will be discussed in terms of impact on hospitals, especially opportunities to improve revenue, in the following sections.

General trends

In contrast to physician reimbursement, hospital reimbursement levels continue to increase. This trend continues through 2012, with payment rates for inpatient services expected to increase 2.8% and 1.1% for hospital outpatient departments.

One major consideration for hospitals is that treatments provided to oncology patients continue to evolve. For 2012, CMS is proposing to continue to reimburse 38 drugs and biologics (given pass-through status) at ASP+6%, the rate for physician offices. For non–pass-through drugs, biologicals, and radiopharmaceuticals, CMS states that the payment rate will likely be ASP+4%, instead of the current rate of ASP+5%. In addition, unlike in physician offices, in a hospital setting, payments for drugs and biologicals with a per day cost of less than or equal to $75 are packaged and not paid separately.

Chapter 6

In radiation oncology, the trend has been to reduce freestanding center reimbursement to become more in line with hospital reimbursement levels. As this trend continues, the advantages of freestanding or private centers will erode. Hospitals may experience more alignment activity with physicians as the cost of maintaining and enhancing radiation technology and infrastructure becomes difficult to bear in light of declining reimbursement.

Provider-based status

Qualifying locations have an option to secure provider-based status from Medicare under a hospital entity. As defined by Medicare, provider-based status denotes a site-of-service payment differential. The practical effect is that the overall reimbursements for services performed in a hospital outpatient clinic are greater than those in a private practice setting. The rationale is to compensate for additional costs and overhead associated with the delivery of care not found outside of the hospital setting. For example:

- Hospitals may be required to meet stricter and/or lower nurse-to-patient staffing ratios as compared to other settings of care

- Hospitals may be required to utilize RNs, while licensed vocational nurses or medical assistants may be used in other care settings

- Hospital outpatient facilities must also typically meet all of The Joint Commission's and local hospital facility's licensure requirements

However, this impacts not only provider reimbursement but the patient as well. In a provider-based clinic, patients may be required to pay copays for both the professional services rendered by the physician as well as the facility fees for the hospital. This may be further impacted by a particular insurance carrier or plan, as patient deductibles and copays may vary based on whether the services are rendered in a provider-based or freestanding clinic (see Figure 6.9).

FIGURE 6.9
FREESTANDING VERSUS PROVIDER-BASED COSTS

Freestanding Clinics	Provider-Based Clinics
Physicians	**Hospital**
Nonhospital entity (i.e., physicians) own and operate the clinic.	Hospital owns and operates the clinic.
Revenues	*Revenues*
• Full Medicare fee schedule payment.	• Facility fee from Medicare.
Expenses	*Expenses*
• Staff.	• Staff.
• Office space and equipment.	• Office space and equipment.
• Billing.	• Billing of facility fees.
• Other clinical-related expenses.	• Other clinical-related expenses.
	Physicians
	Physicians practice in the clinic.
	Revenues
	• Reduced professional fee payment from Medicare.
	Expenses
	• Billing of professional fees.

Source: ECG Management Consultants, Inc.

Chapter 6

Depending on the service mix and proportion of Medicare patients, a substantial increase in reimbursement may result from provider-based billing because of the addition of a separate facility fee based on ambulatory payment classification (APC) rates for Medicare and facility fees for Medicaid (see Figure 6.10). When the reduced professional fee under the provider-based designation is combined with the APC payment, total payments exceed those in a freestanding clinic.

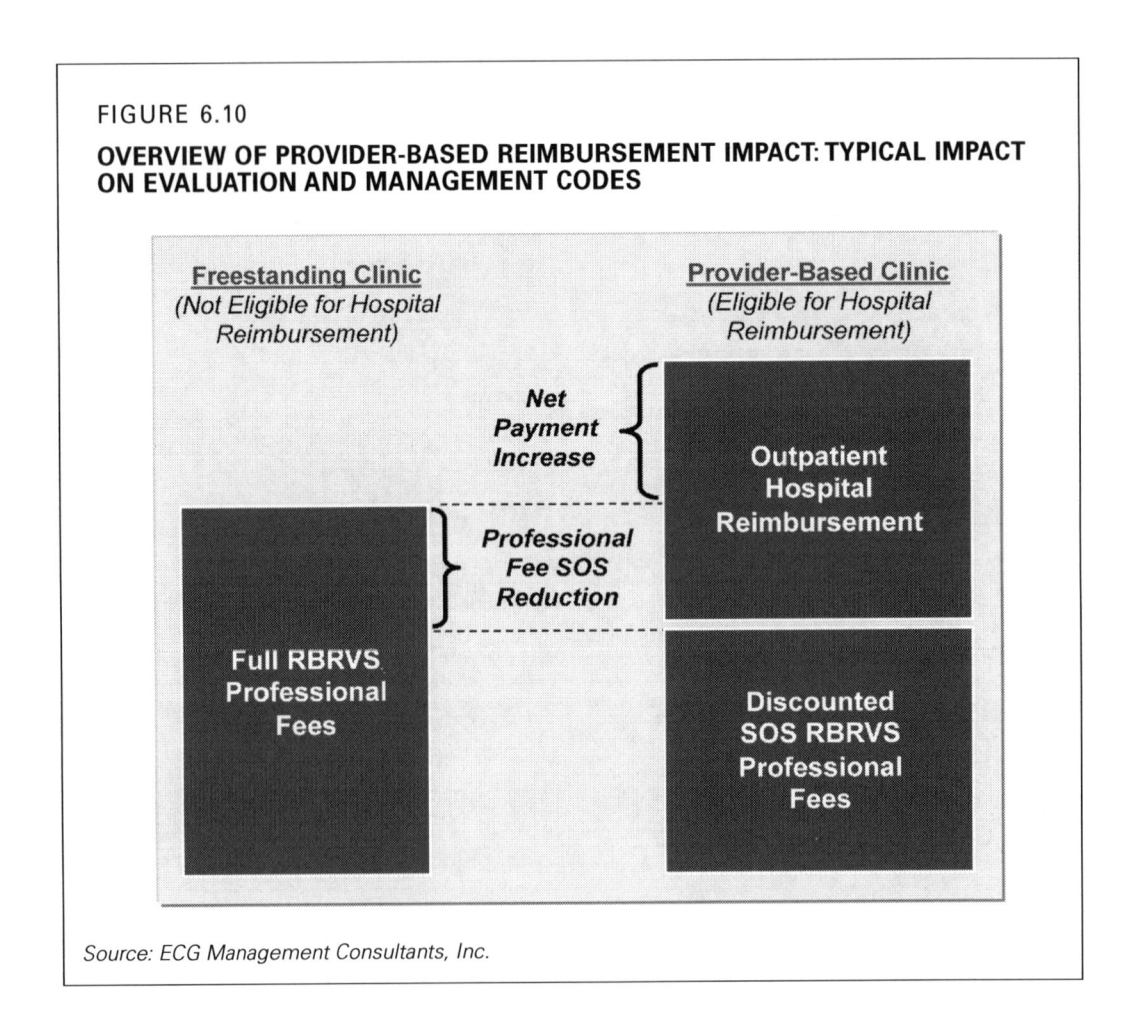

FIGURE 6.10
OVERVIEW OF PROVIDER-BASED REIMBURSEMENT IMPACT: TYPICAL IMPACT ON EVALUATION AND MANAGEMENT CODES

Freestanding Clinic
(Not Eligible for Hospital Reimbursement)

Provider-Based Clinic
(Eligible for Hospital Reimbursement)

- Net Payment Increase
- Outpatient Hospital Reimbursement
- Professional Fee SOS Reduction
- Full RBRVS Professional Fees
- Discounted SOS RBRVS Professional Fees

Source: ECG Management Consultants, Inc.

However, the reimbursement advantages of a provider-based clinic necessitate careful consideration (see Figure 6.11) because they entail adherence to specific regulations and attestation requirements based on the location of the clinic.[12]

FIGURE 6.11
OVERVIEW OF PROVIDER-BASED REQUIREMENTS

Requirement	Clinic Location	Description	Implications
Licensure	All	The department, remote location of a hospital, or satellite facility and the main provider must operate under the same license, unless state law requires otherwise.	• Expansion of current license typically required • Process varies by state
Clinical integration	All	Clinical services of the facility and main provider are integrated.	• Clinic oversight under the purview of hospital medical staff/committees • Reporting relationships up through the hospital • Integration of medical records
Public awareness	All	The provider-based entity is held out to the public and other payers as part of the main provider.	• May require changes to facility identification and signage
Financial integration	All	The financial operations of the facility are fully integrated within the financial systems of the main provider.	• Inclusion in main provider's financial reports • Reporting of revenue and cost on the cost report • Integration comparable to other departments within the main provider

Chapter 6

FIGURE 6.11
OVERVIEW OF PROVIDER-BASED REQUIREMENTS (CONT.)

Requirement	Clinic Location	Description	Implications
Geographic location	All	The facility and main provider are located on the same campus or can demonstrate that they serve the same patient population	• On-campus is defined as 250 yards from main provider • Off-campus is defined as within 35 miles, with demonstrated integration, and serving the same patient population*
Administration and supervision	Off-campus	The reporting relationship between off-campus clinics and the main provider must have the same frequency, intensity, and level of accountability that exist in relationships between the main provider and its departments	• Employees of the provider-based clinic will need to be employed by the main provider • Management reporting relationships may need to be clarified or formalized
Management contracts	Off-campus	Off-campus facilities that meet all of the above requirements but are operated under management contracts must also meet additional requirements	• Staff employment • Management reporting relationships • Facility and equipment lease arrangements

FIGURE 6.11
OVERVIEW OF PROVIDER-BASED REQUIREMENTS (CONT.)

Requirement	Clinic Location	Description	Implications
Joint ventures	Off-campus	Provider-based status for off-campus clinics is not available to joint ventures	• Existing joint venture arrangements must be recharacterized to give main provider ownership and control • Does not prohibit joint support of provider-based facilities • Compensation arrangements, funds flow, and risk sharing can be incorporated to promote productivity and cost-effective behavior
Ownership and control	Off-campus	Off-campus clinics must be operated under the ownership and control of the main provider	• May necessitate leases for assets that were previously shared • Specifically prohibits joint ventures • Requires characterization of provider-based governing bodies as "affiliation committees"

*Despite this regulation, some facilities (e.g., AMCs serving an entire state or region) beyond 35 miles from the main facility may qualify for provider-based status.

Source: ECG Management Consultants, Inc.

Chapter 6

Despite these requirements, the reasons for converting a clinic to provider-based status are often compelling, as shown in Figure 6.12.

FIGURE 6.12
KEY ADVANTAGES/DISADVANTAGES OF PROVIDER-BASED STATUS

Financial Impact	Operational Alignment	Strategic Opportunity
Key Advantages		
• Potential increase in net Medicare reimbursement to the system. • Potential increase in commercial reimbursement.	• More closely align hospital and physician operations. • Provide higher skill level of staffing ratios. • Allow for streamlined ancillary services.	• Convert specific service line/subspecialty area. • Provide funds to departments through decreased clinical expenses.
Commonly Cited Disadvantages		
• Hospital administrative requirements may result in cumbersome processes that add cost and decrease efficiency.	• Physicians may feel they have little or no control over the management of clinic operations. • Hospital-based billing model may add complexity due to registration requirements and IT constraints.	• Hospital/physician relations may become strained by conflicts over revenue and cost alignment frameworks. • Patient confusion/dissatisfaction from additional copay.

Source: ECG Management Consultants, Inc.

Additionally, while the term "provider-based" is specific to Medicare, many commercial payers may offer a similar site-of-service payment differential for a particular set of codes or specialties, potentially further enhancing the financial benefit of converting. In oncology, hospital contracts may offer significant advantages to the contracting position of the private practice entity (see Figure 6.13).

Navigating the Challenges of Oncology Reimbursement

FIGURE 6.13
TYPICAL FINANCIAL IMPACT OF PROVIDER-BASED STATUS

Services	Physician Reimbursement	Hospital Reimbursement	Combined Impact	Notes
Evaluation and Management	⬇	⬆	⬆	Physician no longer receives PE RVU payment.
Drug Administration	⬇	⬆	⬆	Drug administration bundled with hospital APC payment.
Drugs	⬇	⬆	⬌	Reimbursement for drugs remains unchanged; however, acquisition costs may be lower for the hospital.
Procedures	⬇	⬆	⬆	Physician no longer receives PE RVU payment.
Advanced Imaging	⬌	⬌	⬇	Slight decrease in overall reimbursement. Payments for performing advanced imaging were capped to OPPS payment levels whether performed in physician office or hospital. This does not apply, however, to professional fees for the interpretation of the images.
Lab	⬌	⬌	⬌	Reimbursement for labs remains unchanged.
Overall Impact	⬇	⬆	⬆	Overall reimbursement increases typically range between 5 and 20 percent.

Source: ECG Management Consultants, Inc.

340B drug pricing

Because drugs and drug administration are so important in oncology reimbursement, the case for converting from freestanding to provider-based status depends largely on how drug costs are reimbursed. Unlike freestanding practices, hospitals may be eligible for programs designed to lower the acquisition costs of drugs, specifically the 340B Drug Pricing Program.

The 340B Drug Pricing Program was signed into law in 1992 as section 340B of the Veterans Health Care Act. The program was established in response to

Chapter 6

escalating drug prices and requires manufacturers to sell outpatient drugs to eligible healthcare entities at a significantly reduced price, enabling these entities to reach a greater number of eligible patients. Most private physician practices cannot participate, but various types of hospitals and health centers are eligible for the program. The list of eligible entities was recently expanded (see Figure 6.14), but for community and teaching hospitals, the most common means of qualifying is still as a disproportionate share hospital (DSH). Hospitals must have a DSH adjustment percentage of at least 11.75% to qualify for the 340B program. A list of qualifying hospitals may be found on the Health Resources and Services Administration website.

FIGURE 6.14
ORGANIZATIONS ELIGIBLE FOR 340B DRUG PRICING

- Disproportionate share hospitals (DSHs).
- Federally Qualified Health Centers (FQHCs).
  - FQHC look-alikes.
  - Community health centers.
  - Migrant health centers.
  - Healthcare for the homeless.
  - Health centers for residents of public housing.
  - Indian Health Service.
- Entities receiving grants under Ryan White CARE Act (RWCA).
- Family planning projects.
- Entities receiving assistance under Title XXVI (for newborn screening of heritable disorders).

- State-operated AIDS Drug Assistance Programs.
- Qualified sexually transmitted disease or tuberculosis treatment facilities.
- Black Lung Clinics.
- Comprehensive hemophilia diagnostic treatment centers.
- Native Hawaiian health centers.
- Urban Indian organizations/638 tribal centers.
- Children's hospitals.
- Critical Access Hospitals.
- Freestanding cancer hospitals.
- Rural Referral Centers.
- Sole Community Hospitals.

Source: ECG Management Consultants, Inc.

Hospitals are afforded the opportunity to purchase outpatient drugs for patients at the reduced rate, provided that the organization and the patient meet the criteria outlined in Figure 6.15.

FIGURE 6.15

340B DRUG PRICING PROGRAM ELIGIBILITY REQUIREMENTS

Eligible DSHs Must:	Eligible Patients Are Those Who:
• Have a DSH percentage of at least 11.75 percent. • Own/operate participating outpatient clinics. • Maintain a separate inventory (physical or virtual) to track, replenish, and account for prescriptions filled by 340B versus non-340B patients. • Opt out of the group purchasing organization (GPO) for covered drugs. • Have a pharmacy listed on HRSA's Medicaid exclusion file or carve out Medicaid prescriptions to avoid "duplicate discount." • Organize the clinic to meet provider-based billing guidelines. • Ensure that drugs are sold only to eligible patients.	• Have an established relationship with the provider and have been seen by the referring physician within the last 12 months. • Have their health records maintained by the DSH. • Receive healthcare services for a condition related to the medication that is dispensed by a healthcare professional who is either employed by or provides healthcare services under contract with the covered entity, such that the responsibility for the individual's care remains with the covered entity.

Source: ECG Management Consultants, Inc.

National results suggest that a typical hospital can expect to save between 20% and 40% on qualifying outpatient drug purchases, with many programs realizing a savings of approximately 30%. Driven by these large anticipated savings, DSHs have become the fastest-growing segment of 340B participants. However, despite

Chapter 6

the program's growing popularity, its economics are still not well understood in the market, and significant opportunities remain untapped.

In fact, chemotherapy is one of the largest unexplored opportunities with respect to 340B. Because the majority of infusion takes place in private, physician-owned outpatient centers, these drugs are typically not eligible for to the 340B discount. In most cases, the same patients seen in a hospital-owned 340B-qualifying clinic would be eligible for significant cost savings. This dynamic creates a unique partnership opportunity for physicians and hospitals to bring the physicians' drug volumes under the hospital 340B pricing. Total savings will ultimately depend on many factors, but it is not unusual for savings to be in the millions of dollars, even for small to midsize oncology practices. Figure 6.16 presents a condensed version of an analysis conducted for a hospital client considering the acquisition of a three-physician medical oncology practice. Comparing the group's existing drug volumes and costs to the prices available to the hospital as a qualifying DSH uncovered a potential savings of over $2.8 million, or 33%.

FIGURE 6.16
ABBREVIATED ANALYSIS OF 340B COST SAVINGS

Drug/Dose	Price Per Unit Physician	Price Per Unit Hospital	Volume/ Units	Total Cost Physician	Total Cost Hospital	Variance
Avastin VL 400MG	$2,269	$1,653	861	$1,953,979	$1,423,104	$530,875
Herceptin 440MG MDV 20ML	$2,941	$1,625	339	996,935	550,889	446,046
Taxotere 80MG/2ML	$1,402	$1,196	650	911,021	777,530	133,491
			Total	$8,432,651	$5,607,754	$2,824,897

Source: ECG Management Consultants, Inc.

For oncology practices facing the reimbursement pressures described previously and for hospitals facing stark economic realities of their own, the potential to generate incremental operating margins of this magnitude cannot be ignored.

In today's stringent regulatory environment, there are two common partnership models that have been successfully implemented to maximize the economic gain associated with the 340B program: employment and professional services agreements. These models enable the hospitals to use the revenue from the affiliated practices to provide market-based compensation for physicians and reinvest in oncology services (the details of these models are discussed elsewhere in this book). In short, medical oncologists and hospitals that join together can both do better financially than either can do remaining on their own.

Hospitals seeking to augment oncology revenues through the 340B program may also want to consider another potential partnership opportunity, made possible by a March 2010 Office of Pharmacy Affairs policy. The policy allows qualifying hospitals access to a broader base of patients by selling 340B drugs through retail pharmacy locations. By doing so, hospitals are able to purchase 340B drugs, stock retail pharmacy inventories, and receive reimbursement when prescriptions are filled by eligible patients. Depending on their ability to administer key aspects of the program (e.g., monitoring inventories at retail locations, ensuring only eligible patients fill prescriptions), hospitals may choose to contract directly with retail pharmacy chains (e.g., CVS/pharmacy®, Rite Aid®) or through a contract pharmacy administrator capable of handling the logistical aspects of administering drugs. In either case, it is imperative that mechanisms are in place to ensure that federal guidelines for the purchase and distribution of drugs are met.

Chapter 6

Other Reimbursement Trends

Although reimbursement trends related to drugs and imaging certainly have the most direct impact on oncology services, CMS has also been focusing on broader changes that will have an impact on oncology reimbursement in the next few years. These include the revaluing of RVUs (both in terms of the weights of the component RVUs and the total value of E&M codes and certain high-volume procedural codes), as well as targeted programs with the aim of increasing the efficiency and quality of care delivery (i.e., "bending the cost curve"). Although these programs are not necessarily specific to oncology, they nonetheless may have a significant impact to the overall reimbursement landscape. The following section below provides a brief overview of the proposed changes.

PFS proposed rule total allowed charge

Calendar year 2012 will be the third year of a four-year transition to a re-weighting of the RVU components, namely physician work, PE (based on the Physician Practice Information Survey), and professional liability insurance. While the changes to the RVUs are intended to be budget-neutral, the impact of the proposed rule affects each specialty differently, and without additional detail on the conversion factor, the effect on oncology is difficult to determine at this time.

RUC review of E&M codes

In addition to the RUC's five-year review of CPT codes, CMS has asked the committee to review the physician work and PE for all E&M codes (including new and established office visits, hospital care services, emergency department visits, critical care, and nursing home care). This is largely a result of both a rise in

Navigating the Challenges of Oncology Reimbursement

chronic health conditions affecting Medicare recipients as well as the increased focus on primary care and the medical home delivery model. The goal is to have half of the codes reviewed in time for 2013 proposed rule, at which time a reallocation of the RVUs associated with these codes is likely. In addition to E&M codes, the RUC is also reviewing certain high-volume procedural codes, including some chemotherapy codes.

Electronic prescribing incentive program

The electronic prescribing incentive program was established as part of the 2008 Medicare Improvements for Patients and Providers Act in order to encourage the use of electronic prescribing (eRx) among Medicare physicians. This program provides incentive payments for participants and payment penalties for eligible physicians that do not use eRx. The incentives are expected to remain similar to what they have been in the past, with the program expected to run through 2014 (see Figure 6.17).

FIGURE 6.17
ERX INCENTIVE PROGRAM PAYMENTS

Year	Incentive Payment	Penalty
2012	1% of total allowed MPFS charges	1% reduction in MPFS amount
2013	0.5% of total allowed MPFS charges	1.5% reduction in MPFS amount
2014	0.5% of total allowed MPFS charges	2.0% reduction in MPFS amount

Source: ECG Management Consultants, Inc.

Chapter 6

Physicians must report that "at least one prescription for Medicare Part B PFS (MPFS) patients created during an encounter was generated and transmitted electronically using a qualified electronic prescribing system at least 10 times" during the 12-month reporting period.

CMS has proposed adding an additional six-month reporting period for 2013 and 2014 in order to maximize participation in the program and allow additional time for physicians to comply and avoid penalties.

Physician quality reporting system

Reimbursement incentives will continue to be 0.5% of the total Part B allowed charges for services provided during the year; however, payment penalties will be implemented as well beginning in 2015 (see Figure 6.18). Although it was initially implemented in 2007, the policies and quality measures related to physician quality reporting systems continue to evolve. Most notably for 2012, CMS is retaining all existing quality measures and adding 26 new measures. Of the new measures, six are specific to oncology.[13] However, even with these additions, there are still a limited number of measures for medical oncology (four initial core measures and six additional).

Navigating the Challenges of Oncology Reimbursement

FIGURE 6.18

PQRS PROGRAM INCENTIVE PAYMENTS

Year	Incentive Payment*	Penalty
2012–2014	0.5% of total allowed MPFS charges	None
2015	0.5% of total allowed MPFS charges	1.5% reduction in MPFS amount
2016	0.5% of total allowed MPFS charges	2.0% reduction in MPFS amount

*As in 2011, in 2012 physicians can receive an additional 0.5 percent by participating in a Maintenance of Certification program required for board certification by a recognized physician specialty organization.

Source: ECG Management Consultants, Inc.

Value-based purchasing

CMS has proposed a payment modifier for the Physician Fee Schedule beginning in 2015 (with actual use of the modifier beginning in 2017) that "provides for differential payment to a physician or group of physicians." This modifier will be implemented in a budget-neutral manner, meaning payments for some physicians will increase while payments for others will decrease.

Key Takeaways

For anyone involved in oncology services, it is critical to understand how physicians and facilities are paid, what changes in reimbursement are likely, and how those changes will affect the oncology providers. It is clear that changes in reimbursement have already had a significant impact on physician incomes and practice priorities and that additional changes can be expected, including the following:

Chapter 6

- A large and growing demand for services makes oncology a priority for hospitals and health systems

- Because the majority of services have been provided in physician offices and other ambulatory care settings, oncology reimbursement has not been well understood by hospitals

- As future drug payments and professional fees are reduced by Medicare, it will be increasingly difficult for oncologists to maintain past income levels, increasing their receptivity to economic affiliation with a hospital

- Payment reform initiatives, including value-based and bundled payments, provide significant incentives to provide integrated oncology services

- Major opportunities for hospitals wishing to increase oncology service line reimbursement and profitability include:

    – Acquisition of oncology practices and employment/contracting of oncologists

    – Attaining provider-based status for ambulatory oncology services

    – Participation in the 340B drug pricing program

    – Staying current with changes from CMS and health reform

References

1. MedPAC. (2011). "A Data Book: Health Care Spending and the Medicare Program."

2. Harris, G. (2011). "U.S. Scrambling to Ease Shortage of Vital Medicine." *The New York Times*, August 19.

3. Cherici, C., et al. (2011). "Buyer Beware: Drug Shortages and the Gray Market." *Premier*, August.

4. Based on ECG Management Consultants, Inc.'s proprietary analysis.

5. MedPAC. (2011). "A Data Book: Health Care Spending and the Medicare Program." June.

6. MedPAC. (2006). "Report to the Congress: Effects of Medicare Payment Changes on Oncology Services." January.

7. MedPAC. (2007). "Report to the Congress: Impact of Changes in Medicare Payments for Part B Drugs." January; MedPAC. (2006). "Report to the Congress: Effects of Medicare Payment Changes on Oncology Services." January.

8. RUC is a committee of the American Medical Association that is responsible for publishing CPT codes.

9. MedPAC. (2006). "Report to the Congress: Effects of Medicare Payment Changes on Oncology Services." January.

10. American Society of Clinical Oncology. (2011). *Journal of Oncology Practice*, March supplement.

11. Based on calculations published by the Association of Community Cancer Centers, *www.accc-cancer.org*.

12. CMS defines on-campus facilities as those located within 250 yards of the provider's main buildings and any other areas determined on an individual case basis, by the CMS regional office, to be part of the provider's campus.

13. Image Confirmation of Successful Excision of Image—Localized Breast Lesion, Radical Prostatectomy Pathology Reporting, Immunohistochemical (IHC) Evaluation of HER2 for Breast Cancer Patients, Preoperative Diagnosis of Breast Cancer, Sentinel Lymph Node Biopsy for Invasive Breast Cancer, Biopsy Follow-Up.

CHAPTER 7

Clinical Integration and the Oncology Care Model

More than 1.5 million people will be diagnosed with cancer this year, adding to the more than 11 million people living with cancer in the United States. Despite the prevalence of cancer, the U.S. healthcare system struggles with a fragmented delivery system that for cancer patients frequently includes multiple visits to multiple providers and testing sites with little or no communication or coordination. For patients, the result can be delayed treatment, wasted time, confusion, stress, and less-than-optimal outcomes. It is not surprising that methods to coordinate oncology care are receiving increasing attention. Hospitals, physicians, legislators, regulators, and payers are now emphasizing outcomes management and enhanced quality of care with cancer service lines at the forefront of implementing processes to improve clinical integration and care coordination. Medicare payment reform initiatives and the Patient Protection and Affordable Care Act promote and incentivize clinical integration and coordination. In oncology, the major initiatives include the following:

- **Patient navigators:** Many oncology service lines have implemented patient navigator programs for specific tumor sites or patient populations.

- **Multidisciplinary cancer clinics (MDCC):** Growing in popularity, an MDCC places most services in close proximity and provides a unified medical record.

Chapter 7

- **Complementary and alternative medicine (CAM):** Gaining in acceptance by the provider community, CAM includes unconventional treatment options such as acupuncture and nutrition therapy, along with patient education and services for coping with cancer and its collateral damage. These programmatic elements not only improve cancer care but also serve as ways to differentiate services within a market. It is important to have an understanding of how each of these initiatives can be structured, and in this chapter, the key elements needed to implement these care models within cancer service lines will be discussed.

Coordinating Cancer Care: The Importance of the Navigator Role

Prior chapters of this book have focused on the enhanced coordination required to make a cancer service line successful. Each chapter has emphasized coordination and communication in organizational constructs. Although the structure and governance issues are critical, the key to substantive improvement in coordination is often the presence of a cancer navigator.

As patients demand more personalized and specialized care from physicians, the oncology care model is changing. The role of a cancer care navigator has evolved from a patient educator and advocate to a valued team member serving as the coordination point between surgeons, medical oncologists, radiation oncologists, and other specialists. This individual can be either a trained clinician (e.g., nurse, social worker) or, in a slightly different role, a well-trained medical assistant. In either type of role, the navigator is the consistent point of contact with the patient and communicates pertinent information between the patient and the healthcare team as well as among healthcare team members.

Establishing a navigator program

Cancer programs most often start navigator programs by focusing on one or two particular tumor sites that have strong physician interest. Two types of scenarios that may drive an initial investment in a navigator program include the following:

- The organization establishes care coordination among existing providers as a priority. Navigator position(s) are created to increase cohesion and communication among resources and services.

- New physicians are recruited or a new tumor site/type program is created. A navigator is hired to ensure clinical coordination.

Regardless of the genesis of the program, it is critical that the navigator role be part of a larger strategy for cancer care, with specific goals, a clearly articulated role for the navigator, and consensus among providers that the role is necessary and important. The subsection that follows describes the typical duties of a nurse navigator.

Defining the nurse navigator role

Most programs seek to develop a nurse navigator role to act as the clinical "quarterback" for the patient. The nurse may be interested in the role from previous experience in oncology or may be seeking a transition to the navigator role from a staff position. Figure 7.1 provides additional details on the roles and responsibilities of a typical nurse navigator.

Chapter 7

FIGURE 7.1
NURSE NAVIGATOR: ROLES AND RESPONSIBILITIES

Role	Responsibilities
Patient care coordination	• Serves as a point of contact for new patients through the initial visit, surgery/treatment, and any transitions to the appropriate surgical, medical, and/or radiation oncology appointments • Obtains tests, patient records, authorizations, and other paperwork required prior to appointments • Is present to meet the patient on the first appointment and continues to follow up with the patient as needed throughout the plan of care • Conducts initial nursing assessment, as appropriate • Liaisons with clinical staff to order tests and review results • Documents services within electronic health record or patient chart
Patient education	• Answers questions regarding treatment and specific cancer diagnosis • Enhances patient awareness of disease, diagnosis, treatment, and support programs through distribution of educational materials and access to seminars, support groups, and national, regional, or community cancer services • Acts as an advocate in the community by participating in health fairs and community outreach activities; expands awareness through patient screenings, education activities, and community events

FIGURE 7.1

NURSE NAVIGATOR: ROLES AND RESPONSIBILITIES (CONT.)

Role	Responsibilities
Patient referral	• Coordinates referral to supportive care services, such as pastoral care, nutrition, social work, genetic counseling, and other CAM programs • Directs patients to resources, such as lodging and travel support, to help maintain compliance with treatment protocols
Tumor board	• Coordinates/obtains in appropriate format all information for patients' presentation for tumor board • Creates tumor board patient list and organizes conference • Maintains documentation of patients' plans and communicates care recommendations to patients
Assistance and coordination	• Communicates and coordinates care with hospital services (e.g., radiology, infusion unit, admissions, inpatient unit) • Collaborates with other disciplines (e.g., palliative care, dietitian, social work, clinical research program) • Acts as a patient resource for symptoms related to illness or long-term effects of disease • Coordinates referrals to home care/hospice service
Clinical research	• Screens for clinical trials as appropriate and obtains consent for tissue collection

Source: ECG Management Consultants, Inc.

Chapter 7

Programs often experience an interest in lay staff seeking navigation positions. Additional information is provided in the following box; however, these types of patient navigators can be very influential and effective in the care model.

> **PATIENT NAVIGATOR VS. NURSE NAVIGATOR: WHAT'S THE DIFFERENCE?**
>
> Patient navigators are staff who also fill the navigation role but are not clinically trained professional staff (e.g., nursing, social work). In some programs, the patient navigator's role is to provide peer support to cancer patients. Often, these navigators are cancer survivors who have received specific training. Certain programs establish patient navigators in infusion areas and support patient care activities by having the navigators talk with patients and family members about the experience, enhance awareness of educational and supportive care programming, and act as ambassadors for the cancer program. In other programs, patient navigators fill a specific need as a liaison to a particular community. Certain communities have long-standing cultural, economic, and social norms, and a patient navigator can help transition and coordinate healthcare in a sensitive manner. With this type of navigator, there is a smaller role in clinical coordination.

New Approach to Treatment Planning: Multidisciplinary Care

The concept of multidisciplinary programs is not new—it dates back to the late 1950s as physicians found benefits to patients if care was better coordinated across several specialties or departments (sometimes known as "affinity groups"). In oncology, the model is designed to foster greater interdisciplinary interaction to optimize care and improve outcomes. During the past 15 years, many studies have resulted in convincing evidence that the multidisciplinary approach has improved the care of cancer patients by reducing variations in treatment, facilitating clinical trials, and improving the coordination of specialty care. So why is this not yet the

Clinical Integration and the Oncology Care Model

norm? Implementing and sustaining a multidisciplinary approach to care can be extremely challenging depending on several factors, such as the size and scope of the cancer program, the competitive landscape of the providers, and the organizational structure of the center, including hospital/physician relationships. Despite the challenges, at most facilities that treat cancer there is considerable interest in developing a more coordinated approach to cancer care. These interests include the following:

- The renewed focus of hospitals and physicians on discussing opportunities for economic alignment has led to more open dialogue related to collaborative, multidisciplinary approaches to care, with cancer often topping the list

- A renewed focus on quality and new pressures to demonstrate value to consumers have forced hospitals and physicians to assess and improve their ability to measure, collaboratively study, and improve cancer treatment outcomes

- A new generation of more informed patients and their primary care physicians is increasingly demanding more responsive services, including immediate access and well-coordinated care for cancer, as well as other diseases

- As hospitals recapitalize their cancer facilities, most designs are calling for a central suite of services under one roof, which often leads to the better coordination of care across several disciplines and new considerations for work flow

Chapter 7

- Accreditation bodies such as the Commission on Cancer require the demonstration of multidisciplinary programs

- A declaration that the cancer program is comprehensive is no longer sufficient—patients are seeking evidence of true patient-centric, multidisciplinary care

One size does not fit all

There is no universal definition or set of protocols to follow to successfully implement a multidisciplinary approach to cancer treatment. The extent of meaningful coordinated care can vary significantly from one cancer center to the next. While a navigator may lead patients seamlessly through their planning and treatment of breast cancer at one organization, the structure and physician relations in another market may bring challenges to implementing this service at a similar program elsewhere. Moreover, the task of obtaining physician buy-in and "selling" the tangible and intangible benefits of migrating to a more team-oriented approach to senior executives can be difficult. To be successful, the organization should find a way to bring physicians to the table and demonstrate the mutual benefit of migrating to a multidisciplinary approach. Once this is done, the cancer program can begin a collaborative process, one program at a time. The goal is to have physicians speak in terms of "our initiatives" and "our challenges" rather than the hospital's needs and challenges.

Figure 7.2 provides an overview of the integration continuum for multidisciplinary services. As cancer programs create physician integration across specialties, the level of clinical coordination and communication is enhanced. The patient

Clinical Integration and the Oncology Care Model

experience most often changes from moving between silos with weekly conferences to a more coordinated approach for individual treatment plans, including routine interspecialty communication in a patient-centric model.

FIGURE 7.2
CONTINUUM OF MULTIDISCIPLINARY CARE

Level	Description	Impact on Physicians
Level 4 – Multidisciplinary Care	Physicians from multiple disciplines are involved in the patient's care. This includes clinical pathways and protocols, as well as regular communication among clinicians.	Physicians must agree to participate in the various programs developed by the cancer center and follow the clinical protocols established by the cancer center.
Level 3 – Multidisciplinary Clinic	Patients meet with various specialists in a single visit. The physicians discuss the patient's case and recommend a course of treatment.	Physicians must agree to block out designated times to participate in the clinic.
Level 2 – Multidisciplinary Tumor Boards	Physicians from multiple disciplines meet to review cases and discuss treatment plans for patients.	Physicians must agree to regularly participate in the tumor boards (typically held outside of clinic time and not reimbursed by third-party payers).
Level 1 – Sequential Multidisciplinary Care	Patients are referred from one specialist to another. Preferably, all of the providers (in addition to support services) are located in a cancer center, with proximity to one another. At this level, programs may also begin to measure and report on clinical outcomes.	Physicians must agree to locate at least a portion of their practice in the cancer center.

Source: ECG Management Consultants, Inc.

Naturally, the ability to implement increased levels of integration and coordination greatly depends on a number of factors, including the type, size, and setting of physician service, hospital-based resources, and diagnostic and treatment facilities. Figure 7.3 offers some general strategies and approaches for migrating to a multidisciplinary cancer center model.

Chapter 7

FIGURE 7.3
COMMON APPROACHES TO MULTIDISCIPLINARY CARE

Setting/Situation	Potential Enablers to Migrating to a Multidisciplinary Model
Hospital-based cancer center of 400-bed community hospital supported by multiple private practices	• Redesign medical directorship agreements to include incentives for multidisciplinary program development in coordination with service line executives • Use a facility planning process to bring the leadership of private practices together to explore more collaborative care delivery models • Include a professional services agreement arrangement with medical oncologists and a hospital-based infusion center in the service line • Consider beginning with the development of a multidisciplinary approach for high-profile programs such as breast cancer through colocation of services and implementation of navigator(s) • Spend the money, time, and effort necessary to ensure that a seasoned senior administrator is in place for the oncology service line, with a focus on the development of multidisciplinary clinics in partnership with private practices • Leverage empirical market-based data to demonstrate to physicians the value of improving the coordination of care to the benefit of patients and stature of the cancer center

FIGURE 7.3
COMMON APPROACHES TO MULTIDISCIPLINARY CARE (CONT.)

Setting/Situation	Potential Enablers to Migrating to a Multidisciplinary Model
Cancer center owned by integrated academic medical center in highly competitive market with high degree of autonomy among clinical departments/divisions	• Establish a cancer center board or council chaired by a cancer center director with oversight of the development fund and a central charge of developing a patient-centric, multidisciplinary model across participating departments/divisions • Consolidate the clinical support staffing model of a cancer center and redesign funds flow so all respective departments have a vested interest in the center (i.e., use financials as a means to encourage departments to put the interests of the center first) • Embrace and emphasize teaching and translational research associated with cancer centers to broaden the meaning of a multidisciplinary center • Allow the cancer center director to play an active role in setting the faculty incentive components, with strong linkages to coordination of patient care and research
Limited cancer program at a small, rural community hospital with little competition but competitive threats looming	• Leverage existing outpatient treatment services such as radiation oncology and chemotherapy, and explore affiliation with larger systems to provide access to other services through a multidisciplinary model • Help facilitate the development of more collaborative relationships among the physicians affiliated with the cancer program through tumor board meetings and other forums that focus on outcomes and improvement of quality and service • Engage physicians through the use of standard market-based reports to study out-migration trends and other indicators that may underscore the need for better coordination of care among providers locally

Source: ECG Management Consultants, Inc.

Chapter 7

Implementing a multidisciplinary clinic

Most MDCCs begin with securing the commitment of physician specialists involved in the treatment process to create a "one-stop" patient experience. This one-stop experience involves providing consultation and evaluation services in one location within a single clinic visit whenever possible. To facilitate this process, MDCCs are often built around specific tumor site programs (i.e., breast, colorectal, lung). Surgeons, radiation oncologists, and medical oncologists, as well as pathologists, radiologists, and other specialists, are expected to provide care in the clinic at certain times. The patient is evaluated by the different specialists, the team decides on the proper treatment plan, and the patient is informed of the plan within a 24- to 48-hour period. Nurse navigators and supportive care services help provide the patient with a comprehensive package of resources.

The major draw to patients is that MDCCs have decreased the amount of time it takes to evaluate, coordinate, and initiate a patient's treatment plan. With the right communication support, many programs experience an increase in market share as additional patients are brought into the cancer program. Although the benefit to the patient and program is apparent, physicians are often skeptical. Physicians' major concerns include the potential loss of income and a reduced level of control over patients and care protocols. In short, they worry about getting paid less, seeing fewer patients than they would in their own clinical setting, and being told how to practice medicine if they participate in this new endeavor. Gaining support and buy-in can be facilitated by taking the following actions.

Engage a physician champion to build physician support for the program

It is essential to identify and develop a physician leader for MDCC development in order to secure the buy-in and support of the various specialists that will be needed. Ideally, this role would be filled by a current member of the medical staff who is clinically respected in an oncology specialty with good leadership skills and a passion for improving oncology care. Programs may not have a candidate who is ideal initially in all respects; but, over time, mentoring and management training can elevate a good candidate into an excellent MDCC medical director.

The physician champion is primarily responsible for education and communication among physician stakeholders. He or she must promote the effectiveness of the process, advocate for the benefit of patients, support quality and outcomes measurements, and communicate the advantages to physicians, including managing physician concerns regarding income and independence.

Secure participation from private practice and/or specialist physicians

The perception that successful multidisciplinary clinics are only achievable at academic medical centers or comprehensive cancer centers, where the majority of physicians are employed within the same practice or faculty plan, is common in hospital-based cancer programs. Physician buy-in across multiple disciplines and practices can be seen as too great of a challenge to overcome at a community program. However, several community programs have adopted creative models to facilitate participation.

Most multidisciplinary programs experience an increase in the total number of cancer patients seen. Surgeons find that they are not relocating current referrals

Chapter 7

from their practice into the multidisciplinary setting but are actually capturing new market share that may have been migrating to other providers. This growth of market share often makes "believers" out of those physicians not initially interested in participating. In addition to this growth in market share, community cancer programs are implementing various compensation models to mitigate the risks associated with physician participation. In certain programs, physicians are paid for hourly clinic coverage. Other programs have created productivity-based compensation models and contract with private physicians at a per work relative value unit rate. Finally, cancer programs are also utilizing medical directorships and comanagement agreements to secure physician commitment to the success of the MDCC.

Coordinate operations to address patient access, patient flow, and revenue cycle processes

Multidisciplinary clinics require a unique blend of internal and external program operations to successfully coordinate the patient process. In many cases, a hospital or cancer program will be responsible for providing the space, equipment, clinical staff, and supportive care elements for the clinic, while the specialists will "staff" the clinic. The following elements are critical to the successful implementation and operation of multidisciplinary clinics:

1. Patient access

    - Use nurse coordinator/navigator to identify appropriate multidisciplinary patients, coordinate scheduling, and fairly determine which specialists need to evaluate each patient.

    - Establish referral protocols that delineate responsibilities for both the multidisciplinary clinic staff and the referring physician office staff.

Clinical Integration and the Oncology Care Model

- Ensure that patient access staff have a comprehensive understanding of the multidisciplinary clinic and its related services. As the first point of contact with the patient, the frontline staff in both the physician's office and within the program can influence patient satisfaction by facilitating a smooth transition for the patient.

- Develop procedures supportive of registration, charge capture, and collection practices, as well as processes or systems that appropriately share information between physician entities.

2. **Patient flow**

    - Ensure that all diagnostic tests are completed, compiled, and available in the patient's medical record in advance of the visit

    - Designate daily room/pod assignments by specialist to equitably allocate clinical space and resources

    - Employ an appropriate level of clinical staff to facilitate smooth and efficient patient flow throughout the clinic

    - Coordinate supportive care services to be available within the clinic and at multidisciplinary conferences, including research nurses, dietitians, social workers, pastoral care, and so forth

    - Ensure that patient activity includes scheduling returning cancer patient visits for physicians to limit unproductive time

Chapter 7

3. Revenue cycle functions

    - Understand the unique billing processes specific to the organization and the physicians participating in the multidisciplinary clinic. Develop a billing model that can optimize both hospital and professional fee billing.

        – Each specialist may bill for any evaluation and management services and/or procedures performed

        – Only one facility fee can be captured for the entire patient visit in a hospital-based setting

    - Develop procedures that are supportive of registration, charge capture, and collection practices, as well as processes or systems that appropriately share information between hospital and physician entities.

A typical MDCC relies upon the coordination of the "quarterback"—usually a nurse navigator, the leadership of a key physician, and the ability to manage space, time, and multiple physician schedules in one setting. Figure 7.4 describes one example of organizing a gastroenterology MDCC.

Clinical Integration and the Oncology Care Model

FIGURE 7.4
ORGANIZING A GASTROENTEROLOGY MDCC

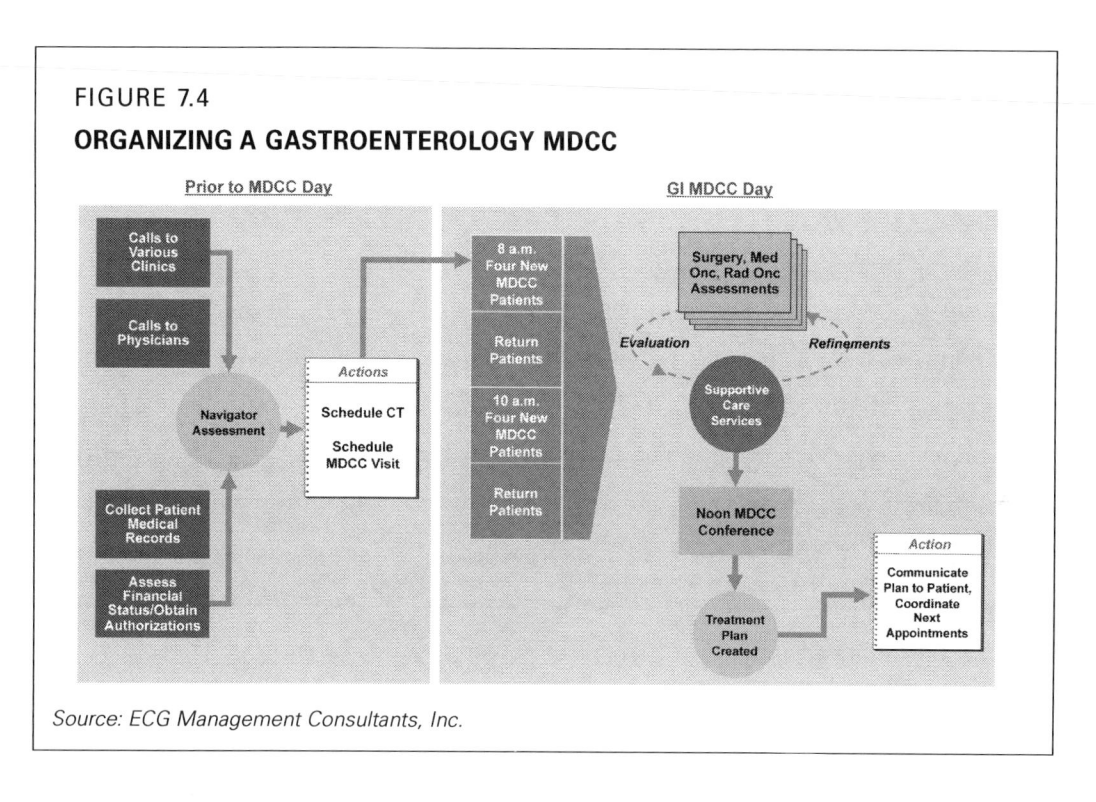

Prior to MDCC Day

- Calls to Various Clinics
- Calls to Physicians
- Collect Patient Medical Records
- Assess Financial Status/Obtain Authorizations

→ Navigator Assessment

Actions: Schedule CT; Schedule MDCC Visit

GI MDCC Day

- 8 a.m. Four New MDCC Patients
- Return Patients
- 10 a.m. Four New MDCC Patients
- Return Patients

Surgery, Med Onc, Rad Onc Assessments → Evaluation ↔ Refinements → Supportive Care Services

→ Noon MDCC Conference → Treatment Plan Created

Action: Communicate Plan to Patient, Coordinate Next Appointments

Source: ECG Management Consultants, Inc.

Prior to the patient's appointment, the navigator collects the appropriate clinical records and test results. The navigator will meet with the clinic's lead physician to review the schedule and evaluate which types of physicians (e.g., surgeon, radiation oncologist, medical oncologist) will likely need to see the patient in the clinic. A process should be in place to support the navigator by having other front-end staff collect the correct referrals or authorizations and manage the patient information process.

In setting up the clinic schedule, the most important element is to create a patient flow that keeps the physicians busy. For example, Figure 7.4 shows four new MDCC patients coming in around the same time, at 8 a.m. and 10 a.m. If the

Chapter 7

patients come in and are registered and triaged appropriately, multiple physicians can start at 8 a.m. and move from room to room, patient to patient. The navigator should indicate which physician is to see which patient at which time, and when one appointment is done, move the next physician into the room.

In this type of setting, surgeons and medical oncologists usually spend different amounts of time with patients. Scheduling return cancer patients in between the surgeon's MDCC new patient visits can keep the surgeon busy and engaged in a productive manner. Again, the navigator is assisting in the clinic by visiting with the MDCC patients as well as managing the physician flow to the next patient. The clinic should be staffed with enough other nurses and medical assistants to move the patients through the process, assist physicians with procedures or orders, and coordinate treatment protocols.

Finally, clinical research staff, social workers, dietitians, and other supportive care services should be on hand to meet with patients and conduct assessments. This is usually a good use of time for the patient, who receives access to these resources, as well as for the staff, who are given access to new patients in one location. The morning of an MDCC day should be busy and productive for both patients and clinicians.

The day ends with a multidisciplinary conference. In this conference, all physicians, nurses, clinical research staff, and social workers meet to discuss the MDCC patients and plan out the appropriate course of care. Various disciplines may manage this conference in different manners—some specialties may want to meet early

Clinical Integration and the Oncology Care Model

in the morning and then see the patients, while others will break at lunch. Either way, the patients are discussed, protocols and clinical research trials are evaluated, and then the plan is communicated to the group. The navigator will take the treatment plan back to the patient, follow up with any questions or concerns, and organize the transition to a specific treatment or modality area.

Performance monitoring

Performance measures should be adapted to correspond with specific tumor types; however, the general metrics in Figure 7.5 are suggested.

FIGURE 7.5
PERFORMANCE MEASURES

Measure	Minimum	Target	Stretch
All new patients receive a new patient handbook with information on the cancer program and a financial assistance packet.	85%	95%	100%
New cancer cases will be presented at an MDCC tumor board.	75% of all new cases	85% of all new cases	100% of all new cases
Patient navigator will meet new cancer patients in person and provide card for necessary follow-up.	85%	90%	100%
Next new MDCC patient appointment must be within a certain number of business days.	14 days	10 days	7 days

Source: ECG Management Consultants, Inc.

Chapter 7

CAM

Many cancer programs are asked to dedicate resources to CAM programs. Most hospital executives understand the importance of CAM therapies, but they often struggle with how to prioritize these services in light of limited resources and funding. While some insurers recognize the benefits of certain CAM services and reimburse or offer discount programs for members to access these services, many still are not reimbursable by insurers. Instead, cancer centers use fundraising programs such as annual program drives, philanthropy, and other development efforts to cover these costs.

Making the case

A National Health Interview Survey conducted in 2007 reported that four out of 10 adults used CAM therapy in the past 12 months. The findings concluded that the most commonly used treatments were natural products and deep breathing exercises.[1] For cancer patients, one large survey through the American Cancer Society reported that the therapies used most often by cancer survivors were prayer and spiritual practice (61%), relaxation (44%), faith and spiritual healing (42%), and nutritional supplements and vitamins (40%).[2] As patients seek more personalized medicine, many have an interest in CAM therapies to manage the side effects caused by cancer or cancer treatment.

Often, selecting the right type of services is difficult when initiating a program. CAM programming can encompass a broad array of services and techniques. Figure 7.6 provides examples of various services or alternatives that are commonly evaluated in cancer programs.

Clinical Integration and the Oncology Care Model

FIGURE 7.6
CAM SERVICES

Complementary	Alternative/Holistic	Supportive
• Psychological counseling • Dietitian • Social work • Pain management • Tobacco cessation support	• Massage therapy • Physical therapy/ lymphedema massage • Acupuncture • Yoga	• Image/appearance center • Art therapy • Journal/writing • Music • Visual art • Pet therapy • Patient resource center

Source: ECG Management Consultants, Inc.

Many of the supportive services provide avenues of expression that assist with coping, transition, communication, emotional expression, and problem solving. Patients can channel the stress and emotional toll of a cancer diagnosis into music, writing, dance/movement, visual art, and poetry, while more complementary services, such as social work, pain management, and psychological counseling may also meet needs within the cancer program's patient population. The cancer program will need to evaluate the alternative services and determine those with which to proceed.

Getting focused input from patients is an important component of both planning and managing CAM services. One way to involve patients in the CAM process is to implement a patient advisory council (PAC) and to charge the council with evaluating CAM services. Cancer center management will need to support these efforts by providing guidance and technical assistance (usually with a social

Chapter 7

worker or navigator acting as staff to the council); however, the PAC can lead the initiative to understand what services are most desired by the program's patient population. This can include the development of a patient survey to gauge interest in a variety of services.

Keys to implementing CAM

Incorporating CAM into an oncology program is not significantly different from other new business planning activities in terms of the need to identify services to be offered, project volume for each service, prepare financial projections, and assess risk. The important difference is that services being considered may not be well understood or supported by physicians and/or hospital leadership.

Acupuncture and massage therapy, for example, may not have adequate scientific evidence to gain support from allopathic physicians. However, if these services are sought after by patients and contribute to their sense of well-being and confidence in the program, they should be considered for inclusion. Likewise, supportive services such as art therapy or an appearance center may encounter opposition from administrators or board members as being tangential to the hospital's role. Once again, the important questions should be whether the patients will utilize these services and whether the services will help in recovery, as broadly defined.

Key components for implementation can be summarized as the following:

- Physician acceptance of services to be offered

- Administrative leadership and board acceptance of services to be offered

- Integration of CAM services with traditional therapies and services

- Services that are responsive to patient needs

- Financial sustainability

Key Takeaways

Payment reform and legislative initiatives have accelerated the trend toward integration of doctors and hospitals, and a multidisciplinary approach has become the desired standard of care for cancer patients. While clinical integration in oncology care is recognized as an urgent priority, progress has been slow. The economic and professional independence of most providers makes teamwork in patient care an extremely challenging goal, and much of oncology is fragmented and organized around the needs of providers.

Within this environment, however, there are a number of steps that can be taken in the near-term to facilitate clinical integration. These steps include the use of navigators, creation of MDCCs, and inclusion of complementary, alternative, and supportive services within the oncology program. In each of these initiatives, the most important ingredient is physician acceptance and leadership. In the longer term, it is likely that greater economic integration of providers and movement away from fee-for-service reimbursement will remove major barriers to clinical coordination and make oncology a service characterized by clinical teams focusing on the needs of patients.

Chapter 7

References

1. Barnes, P. M., et al. (2008). Complementary and alternative medicine use among adults and children: United States, 2007. *National Health Statistics Reports 12*: 1–23.

2. Gansler, T., et al. (2008). A population-based study of prevalence of complementary methods use by cancer survivors: A report from the American Cancer Society's studies of cancer survivors. *Cancer 113* (5): 1048–1057.

CHAPTER 8

Academic Cancer Centers

Academic medical centers (AMC) play a unique role in the fight against cancer. The tripartite mission of education, research, and clinical care has led to remarkable advances in the diagnosis and treatment of cancer. Does this mean that all academic cancer centers, including the 66 National Cancer Institute (NCI)-designated Comprehensive Cancer Centers, are exempt from the discussion about enhancing the care delivery model and organizational design? Not at all. In fact, due to several converging market factors, including pressure to demonstrate quality of care, payment reform, declines in research funding, and consolidation of the provider market, there has been a renewed focus on the clinical and financial integration of oncology programs within AMCs. For this discussion, "academic cancer centers" refer to a broad base of more than 200 organizations, from the NCI-designated centers to oncology programs based in primary teaching hospitals of independent AMCs.

While research and its training programs may distinguish an academic cancer center, clinical revenue continues to be the economic engine that supports cancer program growth and development. As nonacademic cancer centers have become more competitive and aggressive in terms of comprehensive service offerings and program scope (e.g., Cancer Treatment Centers of America) and premier academic cancer centers have expanded their affiliated network nationally (e.g., The University of

Chapter 8

Texas MD Anderson Cancer Center), most academic cancer centers are reexamining opportunities to improve the patient experience and efficiency of care.

But developing a more integrated clinical oncology program is challenging for academic cancer centers. While each academic cancer center is unique, those with clinical programs fall into two basic organizational structures: freestanding and matrix. Freestanding academic cancer centers are not part of a larger organization and have their own administration. Although they may have an academic affiliation, they are administratively and financially independent.[1] Examples include Memorial Sloan-Kettering Cancer Center, Fox Chase Cancer Center, Dana-Farber Cancer Center, and St. Jude Children's Research Hospital. Matrix academic cancer centers, which are more common, reside within or are closely affiliated with a university and have various relationships with affiliated teaching hospitals and physician organizations.

The remainder of this chapter will focus on matrix academic cancer centers and the challenges of connecting and aligning the interests of the school of medicine (SOM), teaching hospital, faculty group practice (FGP), and increasingly, community physicians.

Three Game Changers for Academic Cancer Centers

According to *U.S. News & World Report* (2011), 19 of the top 20 cancer centers in the country are based in or have close affiliations with an AMC. The high ranking of AMC-based programs is largely due to their reputation as leaders in research, training, and quality of specialized cancer care. Nonetheless, competition is increasing rapidly among academic cancer centers and between academic and community cancer centers. Academic centers will need to anticipate and respond to evolving market forces that will impact cancer programs nationally. The following are three major market factors.

1. Clinical integration between teaching and physician organizations

Most AMCs have revisited, or will soon revisit, the level of clinical integration between the teaching hospital, the FGP, and other affiliated physician organizations. All the stakeholders agree that traditional departmental "silos" are a barrier to needed collaboration among oncology specialists, but there is considerable resistance to sharing control at the clinical level. Accountable care organizations and value-based payment reform (while not the only drivers) increase the imperative to collaborate among clinical disciplines. Rather than managing a series of medical directorship and clinical service agreements between the hospital and cancer-related divisions, a more integrated model can make improved cancer care the primary goal of participating specialists, resulting both in improved efficiency and better outcomes.

2. Influence of community providers

Teaching hospitals are actively involved in mergers and acquisitions, both among hospitals and between hospitals and physicians. These transactions introduce new strategic, financial, and political dynamics that force academic cancer centers to reevaluate their organizational design and financial model.

Many teaching hospitals with open medical staffs are actively involved in acquiring community practices, particularly select specialty groups, including hematology/oncology and radiation oncology. As teaching hospitals directly employ or enter

Chapter 8

into exclusive contracts with oncology specialists, this immediately introduces complex issues with the FGPs that may provide similar services. Potential conflicts between nonacademic and academic physicians involve leadership roles in the hospital-based cancer service line, a perception of compensation inequity, and resistance to share the practice infrastructure. Academic cancer centers should adopt hybrid structures that invite community physicians, as well as clinical researchers, to participate in a cancer center that balances clinical, academic, and financial interests.

In addition to the challenge of incorporating hospital-employed (formerly community) physicians into the academic cancer center, there are issues when the teaching hospital affiliates with one or more community hospitals that offer cancer care. Increasingly, major AMCs are forming strategic alliances or merging with community hospitals. For cornerstone service lines such as cancer, this introduces issues regarding the distribution of resources across multiple sites beyond the flagship hospital, including the deployment of physicians, residents, and clinical assets. The jurisdiction of the academic cancer center tends to be called into question, particularly for remote community-based cancer centers in the system.

3. Recruitment and retention of oncology specialists

Academic cancer centers are no longer competing for talent only with their academic peers. Physician recruitment and retention has become highly competitive and costly as demand for services increases and projected physician supply falls. Between 2005 and 2020, there will be a 14.5% increase in the supply of oncologists and a 55.8% increase in demand, leaving a gap of approximately 4,000 oncologists, which is equivalent to 26% of the projected demand for medical oncologists in 2020. Including economic factors, a 36% shortfall of oncologists is projected.[2] This competition for talent is further complicated for academic cancer

Academic Cancer Centers

centers because they need clinically focused physicians who also are interested in training residents and conducting clinical research. With the focus on clinical productivity, recruiting these physicians is becoming a challenge, and it is increasingly difficult for AMCs to obtain funding to support protected time for teaching and research. At the same time that shortages are driving up compensation for oncology specialists, the AMCs are facing decreases in the funding available to support faculty members.

Keys to Success in Academic Oncology

In light of the evolving academic oncology marketplace, there are two fundamental requirements for an academic cancer center to be strategically and financially:

- **Streamlined governance and leadership:** Clear lines of administrative and policy-setting authority are needed in order to make timely, market-based decisions that may have implications for the SOM, physician organizations, and teaching hospitals

- **Alignment of financial interests:** An equitable "all funds" approach that effectively shares in the financial risk and rewards of all participating entities/departments is imperative, beginning with clinical activity but extending to research, as appropriate

The remaining sections of this chapter explore each of these areas and related elements in greater depth and provide insight about emerging models.

Chapter 8

> **NCI DESIGNATION: WHAT DOES IT MEAN?**
>
> Designation from the NCI is almost exclusively determined by the size, depth, and success of the cancer center's research programs. NCI-designated cancer centers are characterized by scientific excellence and the capability to integrate a diversity of research approaches to focus on the cause of and cure for cancer. NCI recognizes two types of centers—Cancer Centers and Comprehensive Cancer Centers—based on the type of grant received. There is no difference in the quality of patient care provided by Cancer Centers and Comprehensive Cancer Centers. There are a total of 66 NCI-designated Cancer Centers; 59 of the centers provide care to patients. Of the 66 NCI-designated centers, 44 are Comprehensive Cancer Centers. Seven Cancer Centers conduct only laboratory research and do not provide patient care.

Streamlined Leadership Structure

Regardless of whether a cancer center is part of a midsized community-based AMC or a major research-intensive AMC, it will not remain competitive unless an effective and empowered leadership structure is in place. The major challenge is creating oncology leadership with authority to direct the cancer center without undermining the role of the participating academic department chairs. A nonacademic cancer program can maintain accreditation and be led by a center director (who may be a hospital-employed physician or community physician) with a relatively simple committee structure with key stakeholders who are physicians and hospital administration. By contrast, an AMC must balance the interests and participation of a wide array of stakeholders that can include the following:

- Chairs and division chiefs of academic departments of both the SOM and affiliated FGP

Academic Cancer Centers

- Hospital-employed specialists

- Participating private community physicians

- Hospital administration

- FGP administration

- Administration of the health science center and SOM

As difficult as it is to balance all these perspectives and interests, the success of an AMC-based cancer program will largely be determined by developing and executing a unified strategy that is in the best interest of the cancer center as a whole rather than the conflicting interests of the participating parties.

While the details of the governance and management structure for an academic cancer center will vary among organizations, highly effective models share a number of characteristics, as summarized in the following.

1. Executive committee/council

Beginning at the top, an effective governing body composed of key stakeholders should be established to guide the strategic direction and resource allocation in order to support the program. Current models include an executive or management committee led by the cancer center director that includes, but is not limited to, the following leaders and/or stakeholders:

Chapter 8

- Dean and SOM

- Senior administration from the office of the dean and/or health science center

- Chairs of participating clinical and basic science departments

- Hospital CEO and senior administrative leadership, including a dedicated senior executive for the cancer service line

- Senior physician leadership of the hospital (e.g., chief medical officer)

- Senior physician leadership of the FGP (e.g., president)

This governing body of the cancer center assumes many different names at various institutions, such as management committee, executive committee, internal advisory council, or director's group. But it should not be confused with the group of established community leaders (ranging from 25 to 50 members) that is primarily focused on philanthropy and which is often called a council. This type of council, frequently utilized at NCI-designated Comprehensive Cancer Centers, is established in addition to the structure that oversees the management and direction of the center (hereafter referred to as an "executive committee"). Further, there are other external committees that are composed of representatives from peer institutions to oversee the conduct of research and outcomes.

The executive committee is not a board, because the cancer center is not a legally independent structure. Rather, the executive committee is designed to provide a collaborative forum to help make informed decisions collectively in the best interest of the cancer center. Fundamentally, the structure is an influential advisory board. If established within an integrated AMC (e.g., University of Michigan), it will make recommendations to the AMC's leadership and board. If not part of an integrated AMC, it will advise the respective executive leadership and boards of the university/SOM, hospital, and participating physician organizations. The specific role of the executive committee should include the following:

- Provides context and guidance for the development of strategic plans in coordination with the hospital, SOM, and physician organizations

- Assists in developing and prioritizing clinical and research programs and initiatives in coordination with partner entities

- Approves cancer center membership criteria and standards brought forward by the director

- Ensures that academic, clinical, and research programs within the cancer center meet the expectations and standards set by the dean and participating department chairs

- Approves the flow of funds related to the cancer center, including the contribution to the center's development fund and reserves

- Approves major capital and operating expenditures related to the cancer center and funded by the SOM and/or hospital

- Approves facility-related plans

- Approves major marketing and advertising campaigns and ensures consistent use of the cancer center brand

- Approves the targeted faculty recruitment plan for clinical and research members of the cancer center

- Advises on the identification of and approves changes to the cancer center's organizational structure

- Appoints the cancer center director

2. Cancer center director

The role of the cancer center director is the single most important factor in determining the success of the center. If not given proper authority and responsibility, the director's efforts to coordinate diverse disciplines will be largely marginalized over time, authority will default back to clinical departments, decision-making will become diffuse and ineffectual, and clinical coordination across specialties will be quite limited.

However, if the position is designed properly with the appropriate accountability and authority, it can be the driver of a successful cancer center that effectively bridges the interests of the departments and participating entities. Although the reporting lines of the director vary by organization, there are common characteristics, such as the reporting relationship to the dean and other span-of-control elements, that reflect criteria issued by NCI that must be met for certain grants (e.g., P30 grant). Figure 8.1 shows a typical governance and management model of an academic cancer program with appropriate reporting relationships with the SOM dean, hospital, and governing body of the cancer center.

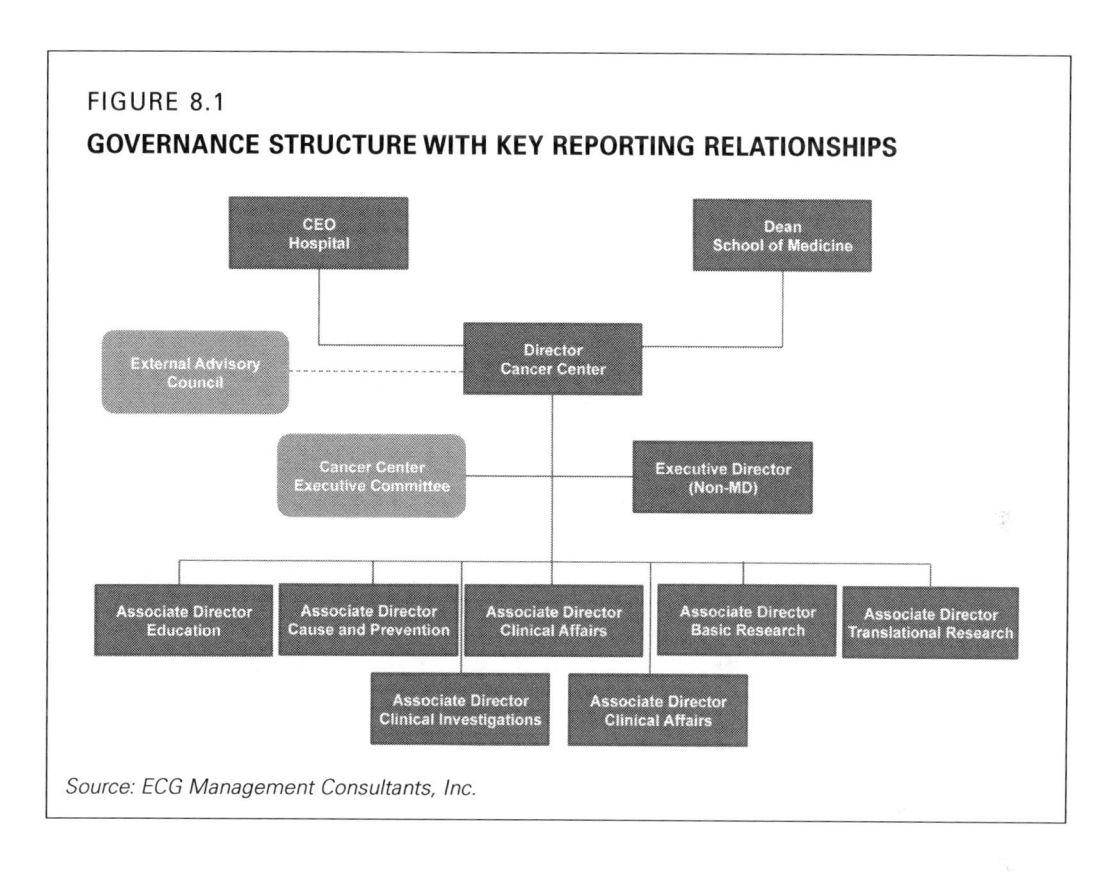

Academic Cancer Centers

FIGURE 8.1
GOVERNANCE STRUCTURE WITH KEY REPORTING RELATIONSHIPS

```
                    CEO                              Dean
                  Hospital                      School of Medicine
                       |                                |
                       |                                |
   External Advisory --------  Director Cancer Center  -------
       Council                         |
                                       |
              Cancer Center            |        Executive Director
           Executive Committee         |            (Non-MD)
                                       |
       _____|_____
       |             |              |              |               |
  Associate    Associate       Associate      Associate        Associate
   Director     Director        Director       Director         Director
  Education   Cause and       Clinical         Basic         Translational
              Prevention       Affairs        Research          Research
                       |              |
                 Associate        Associate
                  Director         Director
                  Clinical         Clinical
               Investigations      Affairs
```

Source: ECG Management Consultants, Inc.

The director is the linchpin to a meaningful and effective academic cancer center organizational model. If the director has authority to shape and execute a unified strategy while serving as an effective liaison between the clinical department chairs, hospital leadership, and SOM leadership, the center will be well positioned for success. Figure 8.2 depicts the balance that must be achieved.

Chapter 8

FIGURE 8.2
LEADERSHIP BALANCE

Cancer Center Director

- Center focus.
- Program-specific strategy and development.
- Center operations and outcomes.
- Reports to dean and chairs (via executive committee).

(Overlap)
- Recruitment plan.
- Faculty deployment.
- Faculty compensation.
- Annual faculty evaluation.

Department Chair

- SOM/department focus.
- Faculty appointment.
- Balance of clinical and academic commitments.
- Reports to dean.

Source: ECG Management Consultants, Inc.

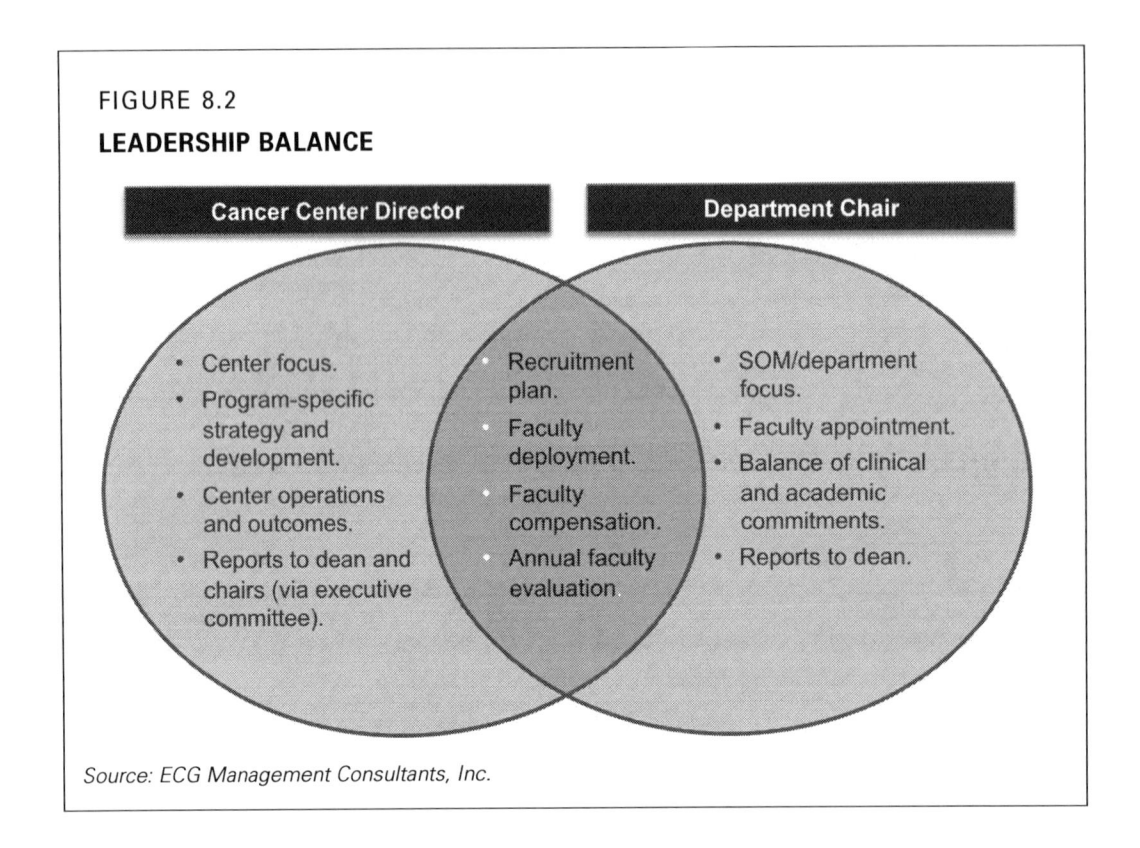

It is imperative that the director have a job description with clear roles and responsibilities that is approved by the governing body and is understood and embraced by all participating physicians and researchers. A director with a full scope of responsibilities and meaningful authority will spend at least 75% of his or her time fulfilling the role.

Academic Cancer Centers

COMMON DUTIES OF THE DIRECTOR

Strategy and business development

- Develop strategies and policies to promote the continued development and advancement of the cancer center in a manner consistent with the goals of SOM, hospital, and physician organizations

- Ensure a balance between and reconcile the clinical, academic, and research strategies related to cancer

- Develop strategies that maintain or establish multidisciplinary approaches to the diagnosis and treatment of cancer

- Develop a faculty recruitment plan in conjunction with the chairs

- Function as the primary representative of the cancer center to the local, state, and national community

- Be an active leader in the fundraising efforts of the cancer center

- Maintain relationships with community providers

Clinical operations/quality

- Determine optimal sites of service, including considerations of patient access

- Allocate research and clinical space within designated facilities

- Determine the appropriate clinical quality metrics to be established and monitored

- Establish and refine as necessary the standards of care for members and clinical pathways to be used by all participating physicians

- Develop appropriate information and decision support systems that monitor the cancer center's performance, clinically and financially

Chapter 8

> **COMMON DUTIES OF THE DIRECTOR (CONT.)**
>
> - Participate in the evaluation of cancer center administration
> - Address faculty performance with respect to cancer center standards and membership in conjunction with the participating department chairs
>
> **Fiscal affairs**
>
> - Establish and maintain an effective and efficient administrative structure and operational controls for the cancer centers
> - Direct the development and conduct the initial review of the annual cancer center capital and operating budgets
> - Make recommendations to the executive committee regarding needed investments
> - Develop, in conjunction with the chairs, an equitable portion of faculty compensation to be supported by the cancer center
> - Ensure that strategic and operational goals are aligned with the annual capital and operating budgets
> - Engage the associate directors and division chiefs in monitoring the financial performance of the cancer center throughout the year

The scope of responsibility for the director and his or her administrative team has expanded in many academic cancer centers as more community providers become members of the centers either directly (e.g., nonfaculty hospital-employed physicians) or through an affiliation agreement. The director must shape and enforce policies and guidelines that foster a consistent standard of care in the cancer center with an increasingly more diverse physician base. New challenges include the following:

- Maintaining parity in physician compensation between full-time clinical faculty and community physicians (i.e., employed by the hospital or contracted through a professional services agreement [PSA])

- Balancing clinical and nonclinical time of faculty, including pursuit of cancer research, in consultation with the chairs as pressure increases for clinical productivity

- Naming associate or deputy directors of various programs who historically have been clinical faculty, but a faculty appointment and/or type of appointment should not exclude qualified community providers from fulfilling such a role

- Collaborating effectively with the administrative and physician leadership of various physician organizations within the same system, including affiliated FGPs and other physician groups owned by the hospital

The ability for the director to be successful does not rest only with the organizational and governance structure of the academic cancer center. Rather, the degree to which the director has shared fiscal control is an indicator of long-term success, as well as the ability of the director, overseen by the executive committee, to affect change.

Alignment of Financial Interests

Financial alignment means that the cancer center must do well financially as a single enterprise if any of the participating entities are to benefit financially. If the FGP, hospital, medical school department, and community physicians are interested

Chapter 8

only in maximizing their own financial position, it is virtually impossible for a cancer center to be successful. Particularly in an environment of limited resources, it is imperative that financial interests are aligned to unify and support the strategic goals of an academic cancer center. This alignment must be achieved at the following two fundamental levels.

- **Interdepartmental financial alignment:** Financial arrangements among and between relevant clinical departments within the SOM and FGP to formally align resources in support of the academic cancer center.

- **Interorganizational financial alignment:** Alignment of financial interests between and among the component entities of the AMC (i.e., teaching hospital, SOM, FGP, and potentially other physician organizations).

Instead of the complex arrangements between clinical departments of the FGP and the teaching hospital and a poorly defined funds flow between the teaching hospital and SOM, an academic cancer center requires an explicit commitment to share in the financial risk and reward of the cancer center regardless of the source of revenue. Equally important is the need for departments to share a reasonable level of fiscal control with the cancer center, including components of faculty compensation determined by cancer center activities.

Interdepartmental financial alignment

Convincing department chairs to share resources for a common goal such as a multidisciplinary cancer center remains the most significant barrier for AMC cancer program development. The complex department-centric political and financial structures that are now typical in AMCs have emerged over many decades and are difficult to change. Historically departmental assessments (i.e., the dean's tax) have been used to subsidize programs or build reserves for development. These mechanisms are directed by the dean and highly variable, and the resulting distribution of funding is not widely understood by stakeholders. For academic cancer centers, an assessment will not be effective in providing the fiscal control needed to drive clinical integration and growth for academic cancer centers. Figure 8.3 depicts a fragmented department-based model and typical revenue and expenses.

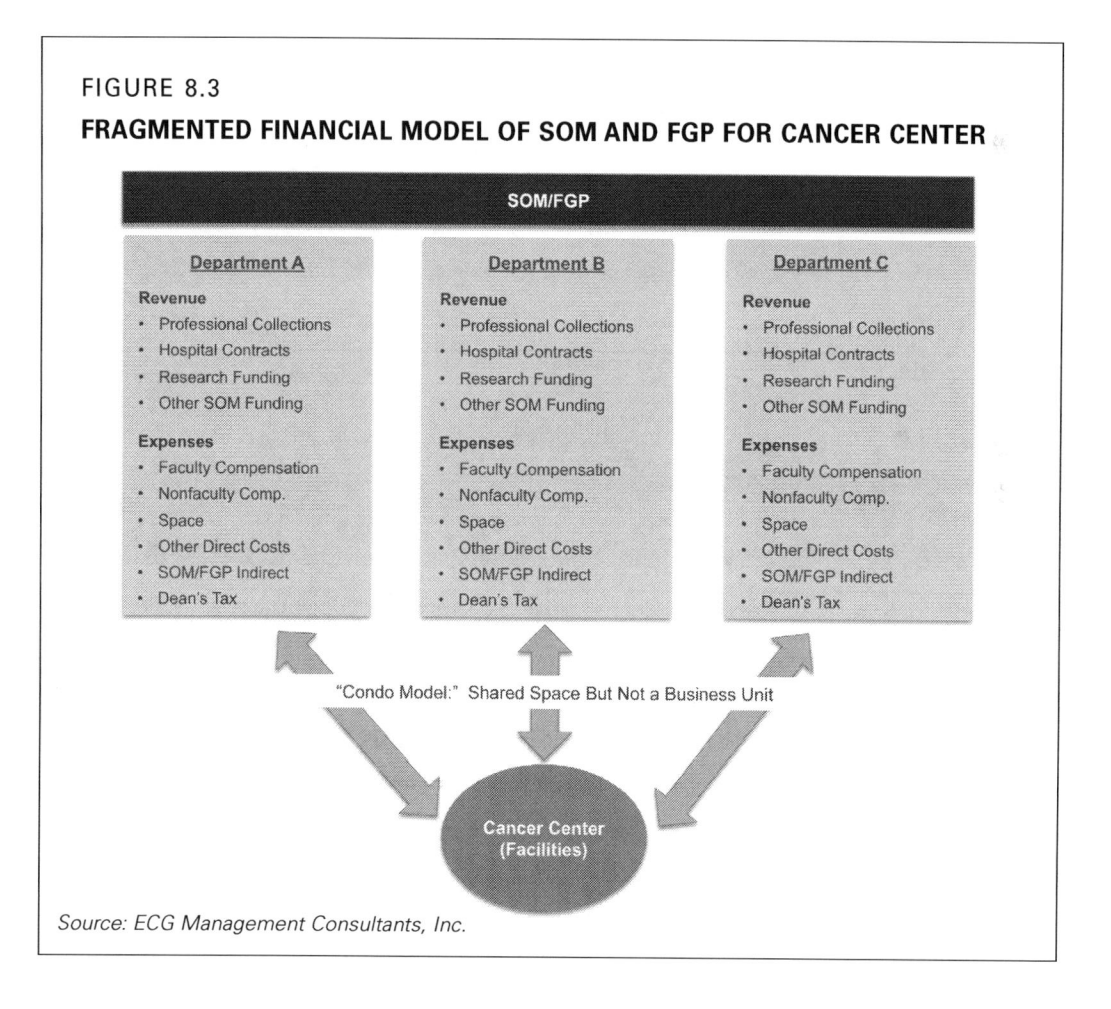

FIGURE 8.3
FRAGMENTED FINANCIAL MODEL OF SOM AND FGP FOR CANCER CENTER

SOM/FGP

Department A

Revenue
- Professional Collections
- Hospital Contracts
- Research Funding
- Other SOM Funding

Expenses
- Faculty Compensation
- Nonfaculty Comp.
- Space
- Other Direct Costs
- SOM/FGP Indirect
- Dean's Tax

Department B

Revenue
- Professional Collections
- Hospital Contracts
- Research Funding
- Other SOM Funding

Expenses
- Faculty Compensation
- Nonfaculty Comp.
- Space
- Other Direct Costs
- SOM/FGP Indirect
- Dean's Tax

Department C

Revenue
- Professional Collections
- Hospital Contracts
- Research Funding
- Other SOM Funding

Expenses
- Faculty Compensation
- Nonfaculty Comp.
- Space
- Other Direct Costs
- SOM/FGP Indirect
- Dean's Tax

"Condo Model:" Shared Space But Not a Business Unit

Cancer Center (Facilities)

Source: ECG Management Consultants, Inc.

Chapter 8

The focus must shift to the collective financial success of the cancer center with a shared risk/reward model with its investing departments. For instance, more favorable reimbursement rates for infusion therapy or radiation oncology should not preclude an investment in surgical oncology, despite less favorable reimbursement. Departments/divisions must become less concerned about their independent financial success and focus on the financial and clinical benefits of a successful cancer center.

Before consideration of hospital-based revenue and expenses, there first must be a willingness within the SOM and its FGP to establish an economic model that shares risk and reward among the participating departments to advance the cancer program. There are multiple ways to accomplish this, but it is important that the economic model reflects the following characteristics:

- Objective standards that are approved in advance by all stakeholders

- Quantitative performance and operational indicators with little room for various interpretations

- Perceived as reasonable by stakeholders, with an understanding that some departments/divisions may contribute more/less economically in the near and long term

- Includes a portion of faculty compensation that is supported directly from the cancer center's cost center under the control of the director

- Provides for capital accumulation over time for funding of program growth, including faculty recruitment support and reinvestment in technology

- Financial performance reporting that focuses on the gross contribution margin and is not inadvertently hindered by the indirect costs of the participating parties

There is an interdependency between financial alignment between/among clinical departments of the SOM and FGP and the degree to which interests are aligned between the SOM/FGP and the teaching hospital, particularly as they relate to a cancer center. With a growing base of reimbursement and cancer center costs residing in the teaching hospital, there is limited value if only financial alignment is achieved among the SOM/FGP clinical departments. Conversely, if financial interests are well aligned between the entities but there is a lack of financial integration within the SOM/FGP, the model will fail. The following subsection discusses the importance of interorganizational financial alignment in the context of an academic cancer center.

Interorganizational financial alignment

Medicare reimbursement policies, most often followed by private payers, continue to favor programs that are owned or controlled by a hospital, rather than those residing in a medical school, its affiliated FGP, or an independent physician organization. As discussed in previous chapters, hospital-based technical services receive higher reimbursement than freestanding sites, and this is true for cancer-related services, most notably radiation therapy and infusion services, particularly if the hospital qualifies for 340B Drug Pricing Program. Because oncology care is predominantly ambulatory, a "provider-based" designation can provide significant increases in total revenue for the same services offered in a freestanding setting. Further, the teaching hospital is often in a better position than a physician organization or medical school

Chapter 8

to finance the required medical equipment, including linear accelerators and imaging equipment, necessary for diagnosis and pretreatment planning. These capital demands are particularly high in academic cancer centers that call for advanced technology (e.g., CyberKnife®, gamma knife, MRI for breast imaging).

The hospital thus emerges as the logical "parent" from the perspective of reimbursement and access to capital. This steady revenue base of the hospital for cancer services is juxtaposed with the declining professional reimbursement streams in an average FGP and core funding support that the SOM relies upon, including graduate medical education funds, state appropriations (where applicable), and sponsored research.

There are many effective models available that can shift the financial focus to the performance of the cancer center and away from the potentially conflicting financial interests of the participating entities. The following are examples of interorganizational financial models.

Integrated all funds model

An integrated model pools all revenue sources and direct and indirect costs and functions as a single business unit with three owners: the hospital, SOM, and FGP. The owners share profit or loss on a predetermined basis (see Figure 8.4). This construct is the most effective in drawing the parties/entities together to consider trade-offs with respect to cancer center strategies and operational goals, and it best aligns incentives for clinical program growth. After adopting an all funds approach for clinical services, training and research activities can be incorporated into a fully integrated financial model.

Academic Cancer Centers

FIGURE 8.4
INTEGRATED ALL FUNDS MODEL

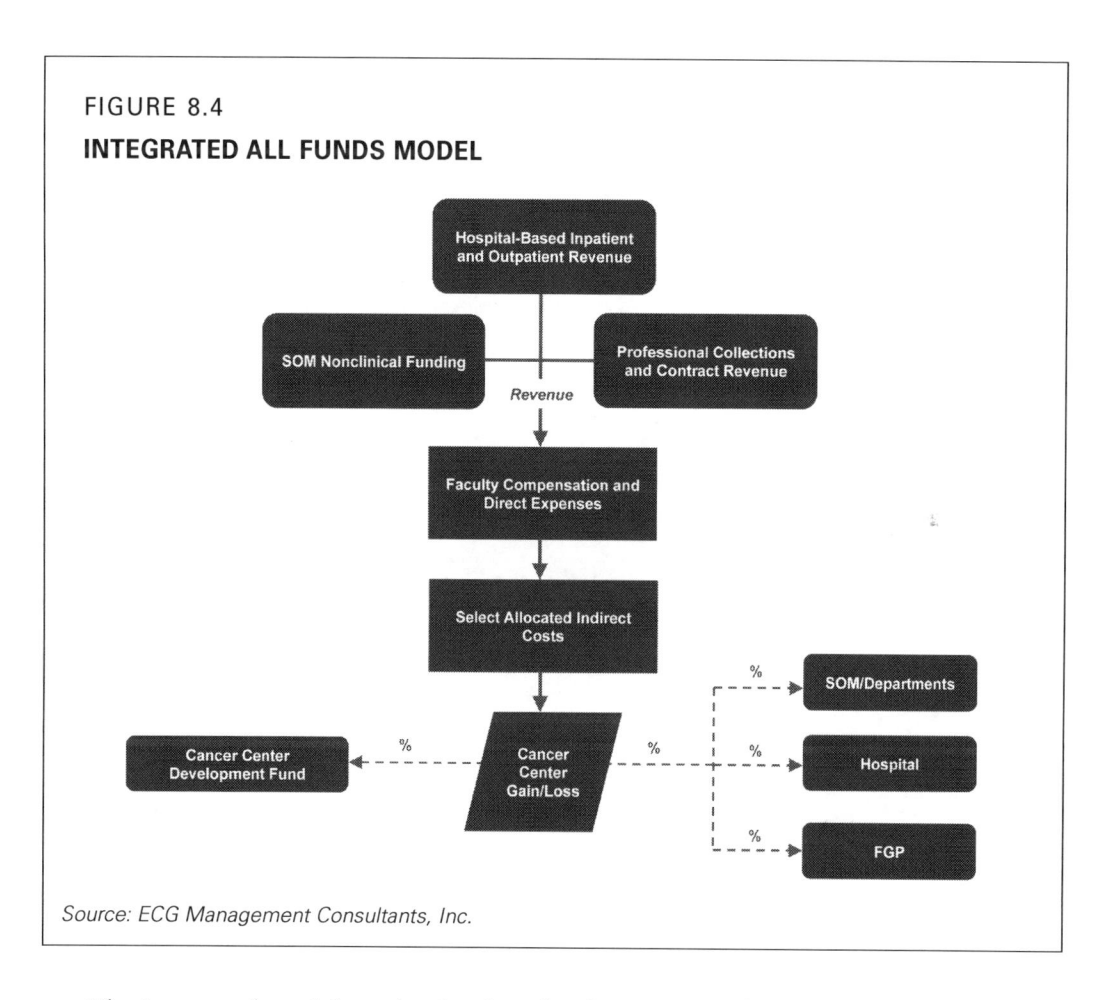

Source: ECG Management Consultants, Inc.

The integrated model can be developed either as a new business unit/cost center or through a shadow reporting system that tracks the financial performance of the cancer center with reconciliation features for the participating party. Regardless, careful design and infrastructure are required to map the agreed-upon elements of revenue and expenses that relate to the designated clinical and potential research activity of the academic cancer center. Figure 8.5 shows types of revenue and costs by entity.

Chapter 8

FIGURE 8.5
REVENUE AND COST

	Hospital Inpatient	Hospital Outpatient	FGP	SOM
Revenue	Payment for designated DRGs.	• Designated cost centers/facilities. • Select CPT codes/product lines. • Designated patient-based revenue. • Technical revenue of designed ancillaries.	• Professional fees of select clinical faculty. • Contract revenue of select clinical faculty. • Technical revenue of designed ancillaries (if applicable).	• Institutional support for assigned research time of select faculty. • GME supervision and administration for select faculty. • Sponsored research funding. • Institutional support for assigned administrative time related to cancer center.
Faculty/Physician Compensation	• Physician salary and benefits of employed physicians (if applicable). • Payment for PSAs (if applicable).		• CFTE-adjusted salary and benefits of select faculty. • CFTE-adjusted benefits.	Designated research, teaching, and/or administrative portion of nonclinical compensation.
Nonfaculty Expenses	• Direct costs associated with designed DRGs. • Allocated indirect costs (if not mapped to DRGs.)	• Direct personnel and non-personnel expenses of designed cost centers. • Allocated indirect costs.	• Direct personnel and non-personnel expenses of designed divisions. • Allocated indirect cost of practice operations.	• Direct personnel and non-personnel costs associated with assigned nonclinical activities. • Allocated indirect of departments and divisions.

Source: ECG Management Consultants, Inc.

Physician enterprise model

In this model, the hospital contracts with the SOM for professional services. Technical fees generally accrue to the hospital, and professional fees go to the FGP. The relationships are well defined and monitored by the governing body, but the structure is primarily geared to build parity between the hospital-based revenue and clinical faculty revenue through a PSA or an alternative mechanism. For example, a predefined dollar amount per work relative value unit can be paid to the FGP under a PSA. This is not dependent on the payer mix, provides support to clinical faculty, and can maintain market-competitive compensation for existing

Academic Cancer Centers

physicians and new recruits. Such a structure (see Figure 8.6) aligns financial interests between the hospital and SOM primarily based on increased volume.

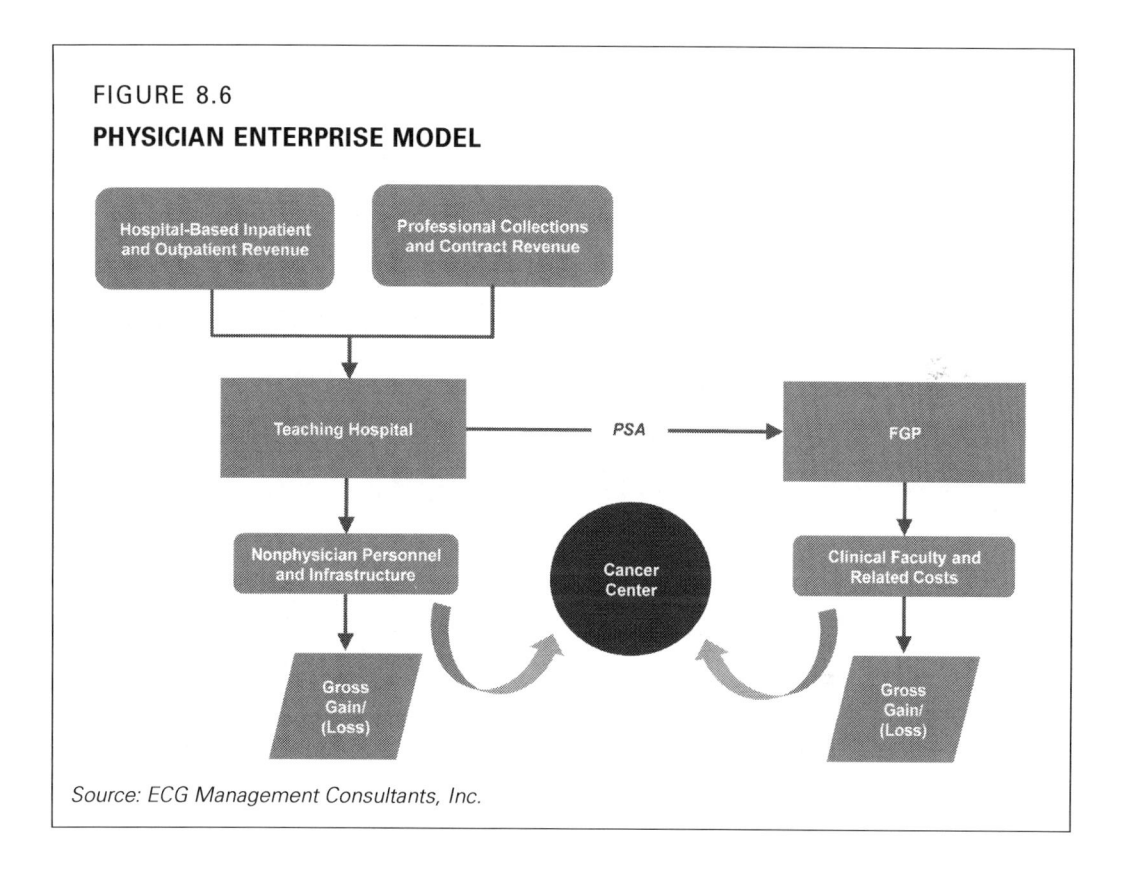

FIGURE 8.6

PHYSICIAN ENTERPRISE MODEL

Source: ECG Management Consultants, Inc.

Hospital contribution margin share

A shared risk model includes splitting the bottom-line performance between the hospital and physicians. Figure 8.7 suggests a contribution margin share from the teaching hospital to the SOM and/or FGP. This type of arrangement is typically based on a predetermined percentage of the hospital's margin, often requiring a

Chapter 8

threshold or excess after a capital fund is addressed. This model is useful in providing incentives for physicians to minimize operating and other costs, in addition to increasing revenue.

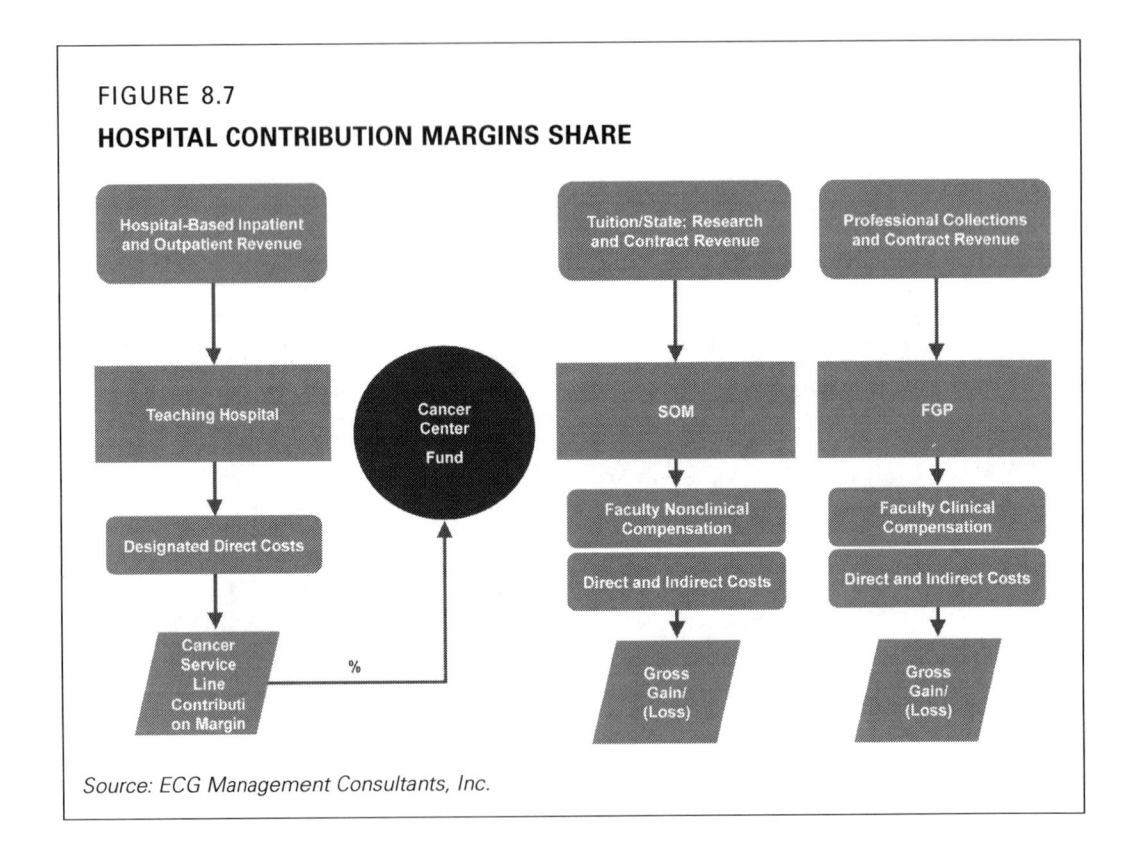

FIGURE 8.7
HOSPITAL CONTRIBUTION MARGINS SHARE

Source: ECG Management Consultants, Inc.

Key Takeaways

AMCs have a distinct competitive advantage in being perceived as the leading organizations for further advancing the diagnosis and treatment of cancer. At the same time, the historically fragmented organizational structure and diffuse responsibility and authority within most AMCs makes clinical and financial integration between departments and specialties, as well as the component entities (SOM, FGP, and teaching hospital), a daunting task.

As pressure mounts on patient care reimbursement and the market continues to demand a multidisciplinary approach to cancer care, academic cancer centers that adopt the following key attributes will prevail in the long run:

- An influential governing body spanning all participating parties that oversees all aspects of the cancer center

- A director who not only has a single point of accountability, but also fiscal control to affect change under the direction of the governing body

- A high degree of financial integration whereby financial incentives are tightly aligned that focus on desired outcomes of the cancer center as a whole, rather than the participating parties

- An adaptive clinical model that is inviting to both clinical faculty and non-academic physicians and is designed to achieve the common goals of cost efficiency and clinical quality

Chapter 8

- An organizational model that does not divide but that further unites the enterprises of research and patient care through contemporary multidisciplinary programs

References

1. Simone, J.V. (2002). Understanding cancer centers. *Journal of Clinical Oncology 20* (23): 4503–4507.
2. The Medical Oncology Workforce, Leonard Davis Institute of Health Economics, 2010.

CHAPTER 9

Maximizing Clinical Research Operations

As patients and their family members become more savvy and educated about various treatment options, it is expected that the most cutting-edge therapies will be accessible through their local cancer center. Patient awareness and acceptance of clinical research has expanded, and stronger government and private foundation support has pushed clinical research activities into community settings.

In 2010, the National Cancer Institute (NCI) Community Cancer Centers Program (NCCCP) was expanded from 16 hospitals to include 30 community hospitals in 22 states. The program is designed to build a research platform to support a wide range of basic, clinical, and population-based research on cancer prevention, screening, diagnosis, treatment, survivorship, and palliative care in local communities. NCCCP hospitals are solidifying partnerships with NCI-designated Cancer Centers and other national cancer organizations to improve patient care and provide patients with greater access to research opportunities.

Community- and academic-based programs are striving to efficiently manage trial costs and revenue while strategically focusing resources to maintain accreditation standards, recruit physicians, and present comprehensive services to patients. To obtain an advantage in this highly competitive environment, a cancer practice must

Chapter 9

successfully manage resources and processes to start trials in a timely fashion, meet participation targets, and limit financial risk to the organization.

The explosive rise in clinical research activities has been accompanied by increased compliance risk. The Centers for Medicare & Medicaid Services (CMS) emphasis on the national coverage determination (NCD) policy for clinical trials and the subsequent focus on the billing of patient care services have complicated the research regulatory environment. As a result, many cancer centers are evaluating current policies and procedures to improve proper documentation and billing of payers, sponsors, and patients.

In this chapter, best practices in both research program planning and operations will be reviewed. The fundamentals of creating effective billing practices with the establishment of internal controls for trial enrollment, billing procedures, audit mechanisms, and quality, as well as an examination of the importance of coordination at the leadership and management levels, will be explored.

Research Overview

There are two primary types of research: clinical and basic. A clinical trial is a research study for the purposes of answering specific questions about vaccines, new therapies, or new ways of using known treatments in people, as opposed to basic or bench research, where scientists and researchers study disease at a molecular and cellular level. Clinical trials are used to determine whether new drugs or treatments are both safe and effective. Carefully conducted, clinical trials are the fastest and safest way to find treatments that work in people. For a successful program and compliance with the protocols of each study, at a minimum, the following are necessary to perform research trials:

- Principal investigator (PI)—Responsible for study integrity and oversight; daily management duties typically given to clinical research coordinators (CRC).

- Clinical research associate, clinical research nurse, and/or CRC—May be an RN, advanced RH practitioner, or an individual with a nonclinical background, depending on study requirements, who performs daily study tasks (e.g., recruiting, screening, and providing care to participants).

- Institutional review board (IRB)—Independent committee of physicians, statisticians, community advocates, and others that ensures the trial is ethical and the rights of study participants are protected. The IRB approves and monitors clinical trials to minimize and evaluate risk in comparison to potential benefits. All institutions that conduct or support biomedical research involving people must, by federal regulation, have an IRB that initially approves and periodically reviews the research.

So why pursue clinical research activities? Generally, effective research programs can offer the following benefits:

- Provide market-leading value to patients, physicians, payers, and other stakeholders

- Have a heightened market presence

Chapter 9

- Are better able to attract patients and top physicians

- Drive downstream referrals and revenue

- Serve as the focus of planned giving and other philanthropic efforts

- Generate an acceptable return on the financial investment

Best Practices in Research Program Planning

Proper planning is crucial to influencing the economics of clinical trials. The clinical trial type (e.g., industry versus federal, Phase I versus Phase III) affects the finances of a clinical research program. Therefore, the types of trials in which the program identifies to participate must appropriately meet the cancer program's larger strategic and financial goals.

In industry-sponsored trials, biomedical industry organizations contract with academic and community physicians to determine the safety of their products and ultimately seek and obtain U.S. Food and Drug Administration (FDA) approval. These studies are primarily regulated by the FDA and may be drug or device trials. Federally funded clinical trials typically span multiple sites, such as the NCI-sponsored clinical trial networks, which are managed cooperatively but are performed at several institutions and associated sites. Clinical trials are referred to by phase; Figure 9.1 provides an overview of the various phases.

Maximizing Clinical Research Operations

> **FIGURE 9.1**
>
> **CLINICAL TRIAL PHASES**
>
> | | |
> |---|---|
> | Phase I | A new drug or treatment is tested in a small group of people (20 to 80 participants) for the first time to evaluate its safety, determine a safe dosage range, and identify side effects. |
> | Phase II | The study drug or treatment is given to a larger group of people (200 to 300 participants) to determine if it is effective and to further evaluate its safety. |
> | Phase III | The study drug or treatment is given to a large group of people (1,000 to 3,000 participants) to confirm its effectiveness, monitor side effects, compare it to commonly used treatments, and collect information that will allow the drug or treatment to be used safely. |
> | Phase IV | Post-marketing studies are performed to delineate additional information, including risks, benefits, and optimal use of the drug or treatment. |
>
> Source: ECG Management Consultants, Inc.

Data-driven selection of trials

Understanding which types of trials have the highest probability of patient enrollment is the first step in reducing administrative costs to a program. Low-accruing research trials have higher per-patient costs and a lesser chance of breaking even. In these environments, administrative resources are wasted setting up trials that will not accrue patients or for which the program does not have the resources to support. Estimations of accrual should be based on the following criteria:

- Congruity with patient population/needs

    - Analysis of the cancer program's patient volumes and community incidence rates by cancer type

    - Historical accrual rates for diagnosis

Chapter 9

- Ability to accrue

    – Physician interest or ownership in the trial

    – Selection criteria that are reasonable and easy to screen

- Availability of resources (e.g., pharmacy staff, administrative staff, PI time) in relation to the complexity of the protocol

Development of a business plan

After assessing the cancer program's ability to meet accrual goals, the next step is to formulate a business plan for research. As part of this plan, the following key questions should be asked:

- What are the total costs associated with the portfolio of trials that we intend to offer?

- How much can we afford (or do we want) to invest in this particular trial, and what are the costs over the duration?

- Should we choose a model that is breakeven, or do we have mission-driven, clinical, or competitive reasons or scientific interests for not doing so?

- How will we monitor gains in market share?

- Will we achieve a competitive distinction by being the only practice in our region to offer a specific trial?

Maximizing Clinical Research Operations

The data that drives the business plan includes estimates of accrual, staffing, and other revenue and expenses. The resulting business plan should outline how the program will focus its resources by tumor site and sponsor type, as well as the feasibility of meeting accrual targets given staff/physician capacity (see Figure 9.2). Performance metrics for the program going forward will be determined by the completed business plan. Structured performance monitoring will be required for the program to continually improve and achieve its accrual, staffing, and revenue targets.

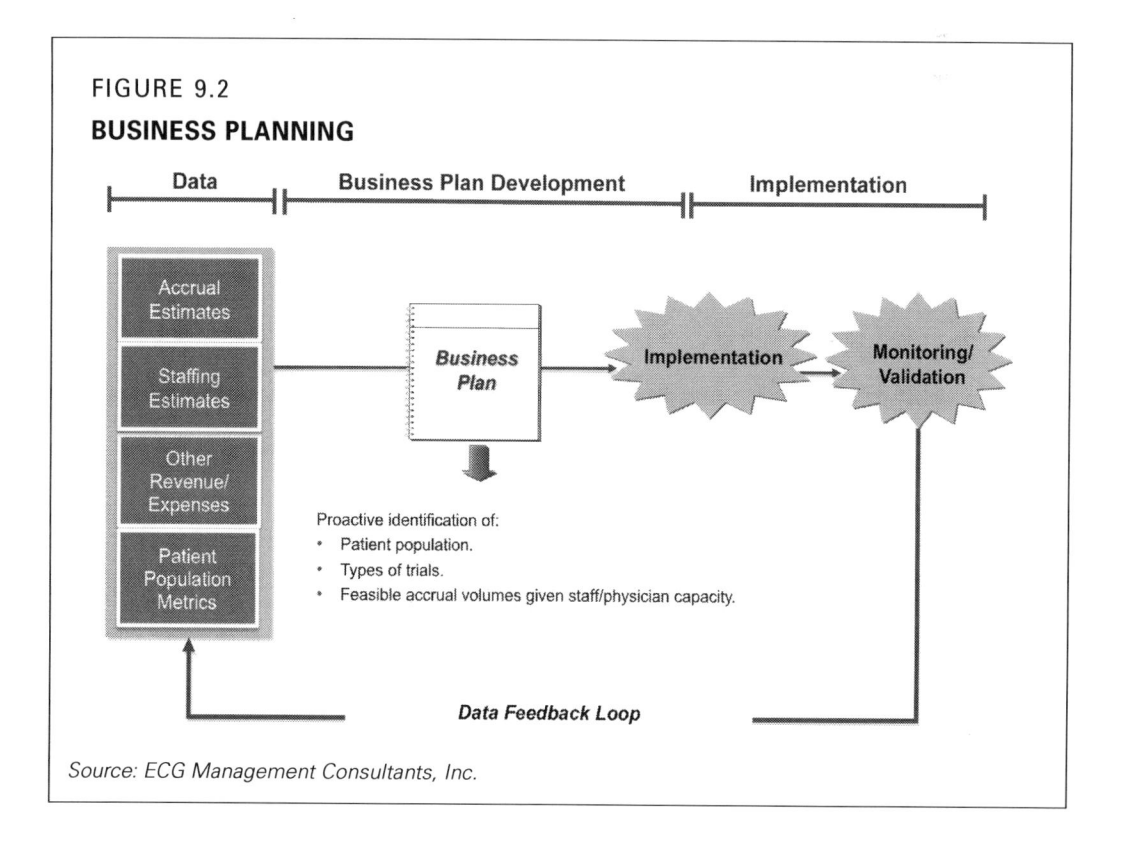

FIGURE 9.2
BUSINESS PLANNING

Data | Business Plan Development | Implementation

- Accrual Estimates
- Staffing Estimates
- Other Revenue/Expenses
- Patient Population Metrics

→ Business Plan → Implementation → Monitoring/Validation

Proactive identification of:
- Patient population.
- Types of trials.
- Feasible accrual volumes given staff/physician capacity.

Data Feedback Loop

Source: ECG Management Consultants, Inc.

Chapter 9

Volume projections and capacity planning

Patient volumes should be projected based on tumor site as well as study type. Figure 9.3 represents example patient and study projections that underlie the financial estimates of a business plan. These projections are shown in aggregate and are estimated for each current and projected study.

FIGURE 9.3
PATIENT AND STUDY VOLUME PROJECTIONS

	\multicolumn{5}{c}{Actual and Projected Volumes}
	2008	2009	2010	2011	2012
Patients					
Phase I	102	98	98	97	96
Phase II	40	26	32	33	33
Phase II/III	10	11	16	16	18
Phase III	12	20	14	14	14
Other	63	74	68	70	70
Total Patients	**227**	**230**	**228**	**231**	**232**
Studies by Type					
Phase I	14	12	13	13	13
Phase I/II	3	4	3	3	3
Phase II	5	4	4	4	4
Phase II/III	1	0	1	1	1
Phase III	2	2	2	2	2
Other	5	8	7	7	7
Total Studies	**30**	**30**	**30**	**30**	**30**

NOTE: Figures may not be exact due to rounding.

Source: ECG Management Consultants, Inc.

In addition to understanding accrual targets, it is essential to model the total staffing requirements to determine whether the program's current resources are adequate given the aggregate number of patients and studies that are planned. Administrative, physician, and RN/CRC capacity must be considered in these projections. Figure 9.4 presents example workloads for RNs and physicians, calculated using benchmark ratios.

FIGURE 9.4
CAPACITY PLANNING

Area	Protocols per RN	Patients per RN	Patients per Physician	Protocols per Physician
Any—Low/average	3	36	105	–
Any—Maximum	8	96	–	–
Phase I—Low	2	20	–	3
Phase I—Maximum	5	60	–	6

NOTE: Actual workloads are dependent on trial complexity. These are general ECG Management Consultants, Inc., benchmarks. Actual capacity will fluctuate by protocol.

Source: ECG Management Consultants, Inc.

It is important to note that these benchmarks are estimates. There are many variables in accurately assessing staffing needs; however, capacity planning is mostly dependent on the type of trial and how much clinical management is required. Part of the feedback loop in the business planning process is to refine and develop staffing benchmarks to be specific to your organization.

Chapter 9

Similar to the deployment of non-research RNs, nurse practitioners, and physician assistants, it should be determined whether trials require RNs or if trained CRCs, without clinical degrees, are sufficient. In addition, consideration may need to be given to the inclusion of other trained staff (e.g., physician, pharmacist, data manager, statistician, grant writer, director of research), depending on the scope of research to be performed.

Financial projections

Revenue estimates for the business plan should incorporate all sources of funding, including grants and industry-sponsored revenue for research activities, clinical revenue from patient care, ancillary services associated with the trial, and administrative revenue for standard program costs. Figure 9.5 depicts a simplified example of financial projections for the business plan.

Once this type of customized template is developed, it can be continually monitored and updated as new opportunities emerge. A budget tool such as this, and the supporting assumptions regarding accrual, staffing, and trial mix, allows the cancer program to track its progress and respond to challenges or changes as needed.

FIGURE 9.5
BUSINESS PLAN FINANCIAL PROJECTIONS

(Dollars in Thousands)

	Historical		Projected		
	2007	2008	2010	2012
Revenue					
Clinical trials	$ 158	$ 395	$ 593	$ 711	$ 158
Clinical revenue	750	825	908	998	750
Total revenue	$ 908	$1,220	$1,500	$1,709	$ 908
Expenses					
Personnel	$1,000	$1,030	$1,061	$1,093	$1,000
Operating expenses	583	602	622	642	583
Total expenses	$1,583	$1,632	$1,683	$1,735	$1,583
Excess/(deficit)	$(675)	$(412)	$(183)	$(25)	$(675)

NOTE: Figures may not be exact due to rounding.

Source: ECG Management Consultants, Inc.

Why Billing for Clinical Trials Is So Complex

Although significant improvements have been made in recent years, the healthcare industry is struggling to implement effective oversight of clinical trial activities. Many organizations have difficulty integrating clinical research with other institutional priorities. In a community setting, private practice physicians and multiple parties with research interests make the process even more complicated. In light of these issues, many organizations fail to do the following:

Chapter 9

- Include clinical research when developing and evaluating institutional goals and objectives

- Effectively assign responsibility for the management of clinical trials beyond IRB review

- Standardize core administrative, operational, and billing processes

- Provide adequate training and information resources

- Periodically review procedures to ensure financial and regulatory compliance

The clinical trials in cancer care are especially complex. Within any clinical trial, therapies, drugs, devices, tests, and evaluation/management activities occur that are either related to standard of care or in direct support of the clinical trial. Standard-of-care activities include services that would take place as a result of a regular course of treatment for cancer care, and these are billable to the insurance payer. Non–standard-of-care or research activities are billable only to the sponsor and cannot legally be charged to a government payer. CMS clinical trial policy NCD authorizes payment for routine patient care expenses and costs due to medical complications associated with participation in clinical trials. Any clinical trial receiving Medicare coverage of routine costs must meet the following three requirements:

1. The subject or purpose of the trial must be the evaluation of an item or service that falls within a Medicare benefit category (e.g., physicians' service, durable medical equipment, diagnostic test) and is not statutorily excluded from coverage (e.g., cosmetic surgery, hearing aids).

2. The trial must not be designed exclusively to test toxicity or disease pathophysiology. It must have therapeutic intent.

3. Trials of therapeutic interventions must enroll patients with diagnosed disease rather than healthy volunteers. Trials of diagnostic interventions may enroll healthy patients in order to have a proper control group.

Clinical trials that fall under this policy must use Q0 and Q1 modifiers on all claims submitted for patient care in clinical research studies for routine and investigational clinical items/services. These two modifiers are used to differentiate between routine and investigational clinical services.

- Q0—Investigational clinical service provided in an approved clinical research study

- Q1—Routine clinical service provided in an approved clinical research study

In addition to the Q0 and Q1 modifiers, ICD-9 diagnosis code V70.7 should be used as a secondary diagnosis for all types of services.

In many organizations, cancer programs lead the way in clinical research. Consequently, infrastructure related to research may primarily be in place within the cancer center. The process is further complicated by patients presenting at different access points within a hospital or system for services that fall within and outside of the research trial.

Chapter 9

The importance of organizational structure and financial management

A key driver of financial success of a research program is a strong organizational and management structure. Oversight of research activities requires an element of coordination within the cancer program and among external departments and should be integrated with the cancer program's other major objectives. Research program management must have clearly defined roles and acceptable spans of control. In addition, the focus of research management should be to implement transparent procedures; understand and meet regulatory, compliance, and clinical requirements; and monitor the financial performance of research activities.

Cancer programs usually start with empowering a research nurse coordinator to assume many of these management duties under the direction of a PI. As the program grows, there is a risk that the infrastructure could become inadequate to support all of the administrative and financial functions. Many programs discover that their operations have outpaced their infrastructure and need to properly realign and reinvest in additional personnel and services to support research initiatives. Cancer programs must be aware of this risk and plan accordingly. As research begins to grow within a hospital organization, the program may also be able to receive additional support under centralized clinical trial functions within the hospital or healthcare system.

In addition to the proper organizational support, efficient and effective financial procedures are vital to sustaining a balanced research program. The following elements directly affect the research program's long-term success and stability and should be evaluated for optimal performance:

Maximizing Clinical Research Operations

- Accounting procedures: Accounting for research trials is different from typical hospital or physician practice activities, with the added complexity of federal versus industry research trials. Depending on the level of activity, best practices dictate that resources should be aligned to support the specific research accounting needs. Standard processes related to budgeting, reporting, sponsor billing and reconciliation, and residual balances should be implemented to support trial activities.

- Tracking of research activity: Although some cancer programs are investing in specific information systems created for supporting clinical trial activity, many still use spreadsheets and manual tracking systems. With any method, it is important to track all research activities in a centralized fashion and to monitor the following: trial status (open, closed to accrual, closed), patient accrual, key dates, trial balances, and other financial performance indicators.

- Contract management: Contract terms, such as payment policies and conflict of interest clauses, should be standard language and negotiated by trained staff. Contract negotiations need to be conducted with an understanding of the costs and operational requirements for performing the study. An individual trained to handle clinical research negotiations should work with the PI to secure the optimal contract.

- Performance management: In addition to implementing certain financial policies and procedures, it is also important to monitor and evaluate the program's performance. Figure 9.6 provides examples of performance measures for financial management of clinical trials.

Chapter 9

FIGURE 9.6
CLINICAL TRIAL PERFORMANCE MEASURES

	Preferred	Acceptable	Not Acceptable
Management of Account Setup			
Budget creation	Within three days	Within one week	More than one week
Time for contract negotiation	Within two weeks	Two to four weeks	More than four weeks
Timeliness of account setup	Within three days	Within one week	More than one week
Management of Clinical Trial Accounts			
Timeliness of transactions	Less than 25% discrepancy	25% to 50% discrepancy	More than 50% discrepancy
Percentage of accounts in deficit			
Total budget deficit	Less than 25%	25% to 50%	More than 50%
Total budget and cash deficit	Less than 10%	10% to 20%	More than 20%
Average number of consecutive months with projects in deficit	Less than one month	One to three months	More than three months

Source: ECG Management Consultants, Inc.

Creation of a trial budget

Cancer program leadership should have a clear understanding of the resources allocated to clinical research and the funding required to support these initiatives, which can only be determined by appropriately creating budget projections for each research trial. A budget should be created for each type of trial, regardless of whether there is funding, to understand the financial impact of each protocol on the overall program.

The protocol, including detail on research versus standard-of-care activities, should inform the budget. The PI should review the proposed budget before submission to the sponsor, and trained personnel should negotiate the budget and contract details. Standards related to budget preparation, format, signature or review process, and turnaround time must be communicated and monitored to meet performance expectations. Within the budget, it is necessary to identify specific personnel costs, administrative/institutional fees, and per patient costs for each research activity or procedure. As appropriate, budget projections for research activities should incorporate both physician professional fees and hospital charges. Standard research rates for hospital and physician services should be set at either the department or institutional level and should not change from trial to trial. Finally, a standard policy should be implemented related to startup costs, defining which are nonnegotiable (e.g., IRB fees, administrative fees, first patient's full cost).

The Nuts and Bolts of Billing for Clinical Trials

The billing process must have controls in place to ensure that trial-related and standard-of-care charges are appropriately accounted for and billed (see Figure 9.7). The major objectives of this process are to do the following:

- Identify the research participant and facilitate front- and back-end revenue cycle procedures

- Identify standard-of-care versus research charges

- Properly bill the sponsor, third-party payers, and/or patients for appropriate services

Chapter 9

- Incorporate audit or monitoring procedures to minimize errors and reduce risks to the organization

- Perform real-time financial management of clinical research accounts

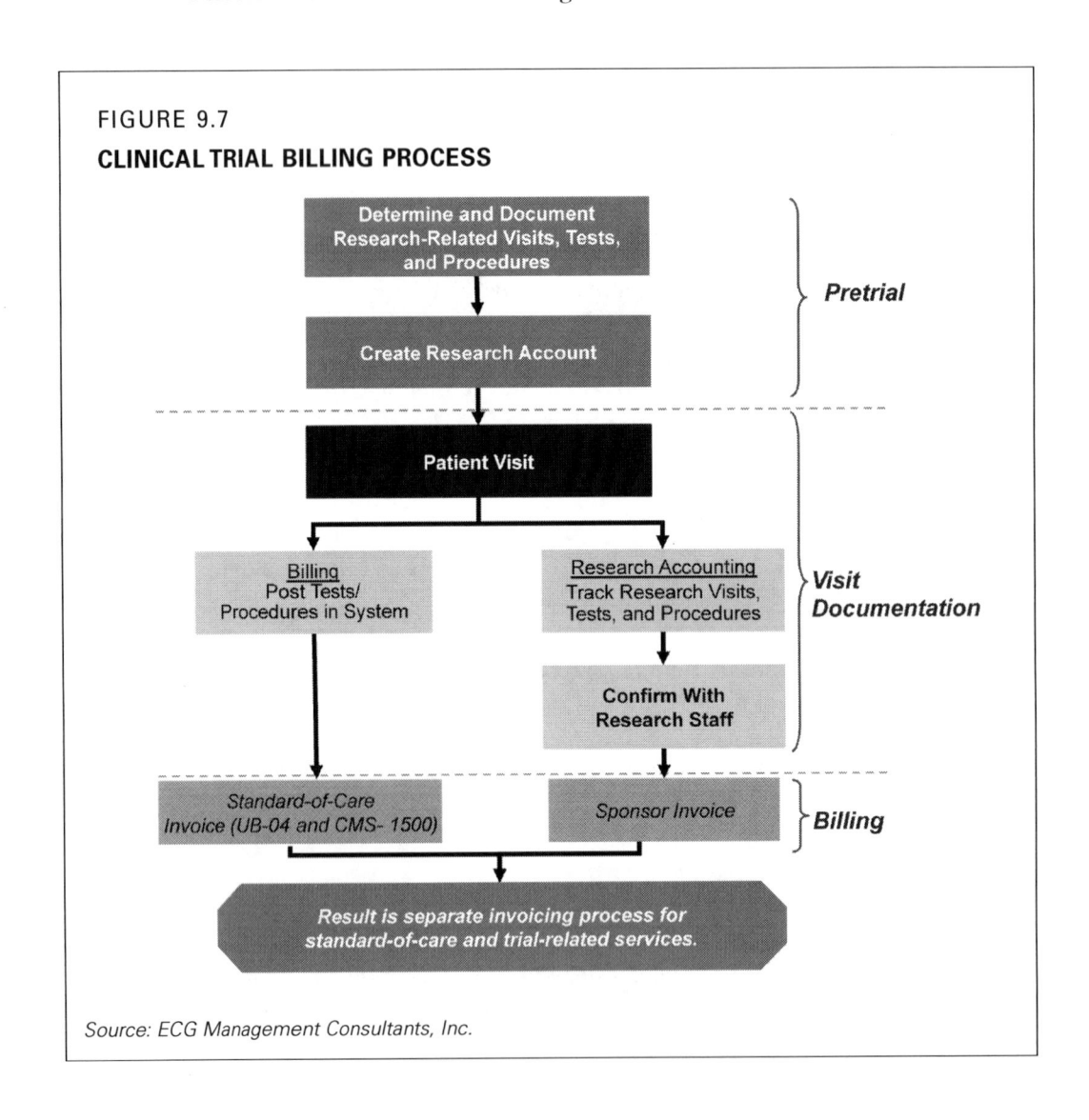

FIGURE 9.7
CLINICAL TRIAL BILLING PROCESS

```
Determine and Document
Research-Related Visits, Tests,    ⎫
and Procedures                     ⎬ Pretrial
           ↓                       ⎪
Create Research Account            ⎭

           ↓
      Patient Visit                ⎫
     ↙         ↘                   ⎪
Billing          Research Accounting ⎪
Post Tests/      Track Research Visits, ⎬ Visit
Procedures       Tests, and Procedures  ⎪ Documentation
in System              ↓               ⎪
                 Confirm With          ⎪
                 Research Staff        ⎭

Standard-of-Care          Sponsor Invoice  ⎫ Billing
Invoice (UB-04 and CMS-1500)              ⎭

           ↓
Result is separate invoicing process for
standard-of-care and trial-related services.
```

Source: ECG Management Consultants, Inc.

Identify the subject upon enrollment and set up appropriate billing controls

When a patient is enrolled in a clinical trial, appropriate and accurate account setup is essential to ensuring correct billing. This includes clear and correct identification of standard-of-care versus research activities. Typically, programs create a specific research card or study calendar to serve as a communication tool at the point of patient arrival or registration. Some cancer programs even separate the research registration account from the patient's normal insurance account by creating different "cases" or "accounts" within hospital and physician scheduling/billing systems.

In most cancer programs, research billing procedures need to adapt and support specific hospital and physician billing systems. At the point of charge entry, clear identification of research services on the encounter form or order sheet will assist in correctly capturing research charges. Programs have implemented systems that use color-coded encounter forms with research modifiers or specific research labels. Others enter orders and charges directly into the patient's research account within an electronic health record system.

Employ an audit mechanism (preferably electronic) to ensure appropriate billing of the sponsor and payer

Once clinical trial activities begin, automatic and electronic billing for standard-of-care activities will likely occur as a result of routine billing processes. It is therefore essential to have proper controls in place to ensure that bills are reviewed to guarantee accurate billing to the sponsor and payer, including coding (the payer

Chapter 9

bill requires unique coding for patients enrolled in clinical trials, such as Q0 or Q1 modifiers or V codes) and documentation.

Although many organizations have instituted policies and procedures that result in careful review of bills sent to sponsors for research activities, they often fail to institute a corresponding examination of the concomitant bills for payers and patients related to standard-of-care activities. This lack of coordination leads to increased exposure with respect to regulatory compliance and financial risk for an institution.

A comprehensive audit process checks the quality and accuracy of subject identification, registration, and charge entry for both standard-of-care and research activities. Depending on the volume of clinical trial activities, organizations that have implemented best practices regarding clinical trial billing have instituted processes that include a concurrent review of bills to sponsors, payers, and guarantors related to the same episode of care. This not only provides a real-time check of the accuracy of the accounts, but it also encourages information and outcomes to be shared across front- and back-end billing staff to continuously monitor and improve performance. The scope of this process is often determined by an organization's resources and clinical research activities; although it is best to audit every bill associated with a research patient, this may be difficult and resource-intensive. Electronic systems can be used to facilitate the audit, or programs can choose to audit a certain percentage of research patient accounts.

Specify payment procedures and support with proper controls

Cancer programs must have a process to account for research payments. Procedures should be in place to direct payments back to the research account. Clearly articulated standards should be stated within the contract to maintain proper controls, such as requiring the sponsor to include the account number on the payment check. Many cancer programs need to work with their accounting departments or grant administration to facilitate the timely deposit of payments. Finally, program management can limit increases in accounts receivable by monitoring account balances, patient accruals, and payment terms for each research trial in standard, periodic reports.

The Last Step: Audit Process and Performance

Cancer programs should implement a regular audit process not only to review the billing function but also to evaluate financial performance and contract management. The major tasks to include in this review should be as follows:

- Review clinical trial contracts and policies related to processing trial patients, visits, and billable procedures

- Conduct interviews with key personnel

- Review process flow documentation related to service, coding, registration, and billing

- Analyze clinical trial accounting, coding, and billing processes and procedures

Chapter 9

- Evaluate charge sheets, research registration cards, and other mechanisms for accuracy during charge entry

- Audit selected research accounts and billing records

    – Include a sample of active and past years' accounts and protocols

    – Compare accrual information and protocol documents to funds billed and received

    – Review invoice detail to confirm that services were not billed to Medicare (or other third-party payers) in error

- Document findings and discuss them with a multidisciplinary group that includes members from each affected area—research staff, revenue cycle staff, PIs, and management (in coordination with internal legal counsel)

This process will help a cancer program stay on point as new research is pursued, the funding mix changes, or the program experiences management/staff transitions.

Key Takeaways

Conducting a clinical research program is complex. Strong leadership, clear and transparent procedures, and effective process controls are essential for cancer programs to successfully navigate the financial, regulatory, and compliance challenges related to clinical research. To evaluate your cancer research program, ask the following questions:

- Are resources available and aligned to support strategic growth in clinical research?

- Are research procedures clearly integrated throughout the clinical enterprise?

- Is budget development executed under standard policies/procedures?

- Are systems in place to identify enrollees, appropriately charge sponsors or third-party payers, and track revenue back to the research account?

- How is the program performing financially?

- How are we managing performance to meet our strategic, operational, and financial goals?

APPENDIX A

Sample Interview Guide

I. Introduction

- The objective of this project is to develop an oncology strategy and business plan that will define the direction, scope, and resource requirements of a well-positioned, differentiated, and clinically integrated program

- The purpose of the interviews is to:

    - Identify perceptions and perspectives regarding developing an oncology service line strategy

    - Understand current relationships and dynamics

    - Gain perspectives on the strategic opportunities currently available

- All interviews will be kept confidential

II. Background information

- Provide a brief description of your educational and clinical background.

- Do you have any administrative roles at the hospital?

Appendix A

- Describe your practice in terms of the number of physicians, specialties, and in-office ancillaries offered.

- Where do you have hospital privileges?

- What percentage of your clinical volume is derived from activities at the hospital?

- Have any physicians recently joined or left your practice? Are you currently recruiting?

- What do you perceive as the opportunities for your practice in the market area?

III. Current oncology services

- Describe the overall oncology programmatic needs of the community and areas of physician shortage/surplus.

- How do the current oncology services fit within the larger system/parent organization's broader strategic plan?

- Describe the nonfinancial benefits to the larger organization from the oncology service.

- Describe the overall strengths and weaknesses of the oncology program.

    – Patient access

    – Growth potential

    – Capital needs

IV. Medical staff relations

- How would you characterize the current relationship between hospital administration and the medical staff?

- How would you characterize the hospital's physician strategy as it pertains to oncology services, including physician recruitment and retention?

- Describe the referral patterns within the service, with other specialties, and with outside sources.

- How would you characterize the current relationships between the various oncology groups? Between the medical oncologists, radiation oncologists, and surgical oncologists? Between the various oncology and oncology surgery subspecialties?

- Has the hospital historically provided all the resources that you have requested?

- How can the hospital enhance its relationship with you?

Appendix A

V. Strategic goals

- What is your vision for oncology services at the hospital for the next five years?

    - Clinical quality

    - Programmatic scope

    - Differentiation

    - Growth

    - Patient experience

    - Physician alignment

    - Research

- From your perspective, what is the gap between the current state of oncology services at the hospital and your vision?

- What are the attributes (good and bad) of the hospital, and specifically the hospital's oncology services, that differentiate it from competing hospitals in the eyes of physicians? In the eyes of patients?

- What would you hope to achieve through the creation of an oncology service line at the hospital (if not already in place)?

    - Increased coordination of care (e.g., consolidated services in common building/location, physician referrals and relationships)

Sample Interview Guide

- Multidisciplinary clinics

- Greater patient volumes

- Differentiation of services

- Increased focus and dedicated resources for oncology services

- Greater physician involvement in decision-making

- Increased clinical research volumes

- Tumor site programs

- Institutional partnerships

- Other

- Are there any technology or facility changes that the hospital should consider to better support an oncology service line?

- How can the hospital best leverage its employed oncology physicians to support and grow an oncology service (if applicable)?

- As the hospital considers opportunities for expanding oncology services, what specific markets should it explore, and how should it seek to attract patients and physicians?

- What obstacles will have to be overcome as oncology services continue to grow?

Appendix A

VI. Governance and management

- What role would you like to see physicians play in the governance and management of the oncology service going forward?

- From your perspective, are any changes needed to the governance and management of oncology services?

VII. Partnerships

- Do you foresee partnerships with an institutional organization?

- If yes, what would be the goals of an additional partner (e.g., branding, referrals)?

    - Marketing/branding

    - Expert opinions

    - Access to clinical research

    - Physician education

    - Clinical protocols

    - Access to multidisciplinary tumor boards

VIII. Closing

Do you have any questions or comments on issues that we did not cover?

APPENDIX B

Internal and External Assessment Key Analyses

Internal Assessment Key Analyses

Volume

- **Historical service line inpatient volume trends**—Charts or graphs showing volume trends by service line sector (e.g., oncology, oncology surgery) for the three most recent years.

- **Historical outpatient volume trends**—Charts or graphs showing volume trends by key area (e.g., radiation oncology, chemotherapy) for the three most recent years.

- **Volume by referring or procedural physician**—Chart showing number of admissions by physician for cancer primary or secondary diagnoses.

- **Patient origin map**—Map showing relative volume of oncology inpatient admissions by patient ZIP code. A range of colors will denote where patient volume is centered.

Appendix B

Financial trends

- **Payer mix**—Pie chart showing payer mix for the three most recent years (oncology-specific, if possible). It should include Medicare, Medicaid, self-pay, commercial, and other payers, grouped in appropriate categories.

- **Contribution margin by modality**—Analysis of contribution margin by modality (e.g., chemotherapy, radiation oncology) for the most recent year.

- **Profitability of service line**—If available, analysis of the profitability of the service line, compared and contrasted over the three most recent years.

Other

- **Clinical coordination**—Illustrate the continuum of services provided to oncology patients, then evaluate the level of coordination across the continuum.

- **Clinical pathways**—Trend lines to monitor utilization of and compliance with established clinical pathways by actual volume, and as a percentage of total case volume.

- **Research**—Graphs showing number of open research trials and the annual accrual rates.

- **Tumor boards**—Description of internal tumor boards, and multidisciplinary team participation.

Quality trends

- **Quality indicators**—Chart summarizing key quality indicators versus targeted benchmarks.

- **Patient satisfaction scores**—Graph or chart showing key trends in patient satisfaction scores in key areas for the past three periods during which data is available.

Operational efficiency

- **Staffing levels**—Analysis of staffing levels and key nursing and staffing metrics for the three most recent years.

- **Staff satisfaction scores**—Analysis of staff satisfaction scores for the three most recent available periods compared to targeted levels.

External Assessment Key Analyses

Typically, the external assessment looks at industry, demographic, and market trends, as outlined in the following.

Industry trends

- **Reimbursement projections**—Analysis of likely trends in physician and hospital reimbursement over the coming years given healthcare reform, Centers for Medicare & Medicaid Services policy, changing care models, etc.

Appendix B

- **Innovative technology/procedures**—Discussion of the forecasted trends in procedures and available technology and how they will impact the provision of clinical care and growth of the market.

- **Hospital/physician relationship**—Analysis of emerging trends in the relationship and alignment models between hospitals and physicians and how they will impact the marketplace.

Demographic trends

- **Forecasted population change**—Table showing the forecasted change in population in the next five years, breaking out key age cohorts.

- **Map of current population**—Color-coded map showing the current population by ZIP code (for instance, darker colors may be used to delineate areas with higher population density). Include markers indicating location of competing facilities.

- **Map depicting population change**—Map showing the anticipated amount of population growth/reduction by ZIP code. A range of colors should be used to reflect the amount of population growth versus decline.

Market trends

- **Incidence trends**—Charts comparing the local, regional, and national cancer incidence rates by major tumor site and in total.

- **Market available service**—Line graphs showing the number of physicians (potentially by specialty) and number of key resources (e.g., outpatient chemotherapy chairs, linear accelerators) in the primary service area.

- **Referral patterns**—Charts by modality with referral source.